GUT HEALTH FOR KIDS

A parent's guide to promoting brain-gut health. Provide
your child with a diet that fosters better mental health.
ADD, and ADHD dont have to be a lifelong burden.

SHEA MACRAE

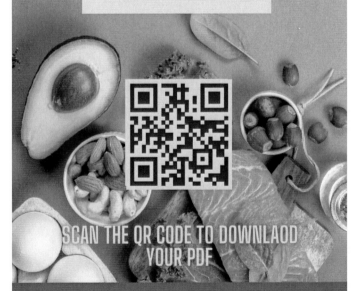

Handy Diet Guide

YOUR FREE GIFT

SCAN THE QR CODE TO DOWNLAOD
YOUR PDF

Introduction

"Your gut is not Las Vegas. What happens in your gut does not stay in your gut." - Peter Kozlowski

What if you found out that nearly everything that affected your health came from the gut? Would you stop to think about the next food item you're going to consume or would this be something you would disregard?

If you've thought the personal health of your gut is a big mystery, you're not alone, as many others are in the dark of the processes occuring in their abdomen. 70 million people in the US have digestive issues, yet this topic is not being discussed nearly enough by health officials or practicing physicians that are seeing dozens of patients each day.

It's easy to dismiss your diet as something that has much of an impact on your overall well being, since many people have heard that 'eating more fruits and vegetables in addition to getting plenty of exercise'; it's been recited as a steady mantra for decades. Most people try to follow these guidelines yet find themselves diagnosed with chronic ailments years after adhering to this 'healthy' lifestyle.

Children are most influenced by your health because they mirror the behaviors and habits that we model for them in our daily lives. If gut health education has failed to reach most adults, it's only a matter of time that your kids will be affected as well.

As a parent myself, I observe how children's behaviors tend to fluctuate depending on how their moods shift day to day. At first I never took much notice of this, as I accounted for this as part of growing pains that many adolescents struggle with.

However as things further continued, I was growing concerned that my son was having difficulty adapting to his environment. He had other symptoms that were affecting his daily life, which is when I had him looked at by our local pediatrician.

Getting a diagnosis of attention deficit disorder (ADD), I was mortified by the potential treatments that were going to ensue to help him adapt to this condition. Prescription medications are almost always guaranteed to be used for this diagnosis, and I was concerned of the potential side effects this would have for my child years later.

I'm a practicing nutritionist and I've always recommended dietary lifestyle changes for my clients whenever I've observed ailments or recurring health issues. My mission from that point on was to treat my son with the speciality of my knowledge and do what was best for his health.

By changing his diet, not only did I notice great changes to his overall improvement in mood, but he was no longer facing any of the challenges as in the past. Managing his diet was not only changing his lifestyle, but it changed my understanding of what may be the root cause of so many of the health problems that many people are struggling with.

Introduction

Through my past experiences and research I want to share with you what I've discovered as an attentive parent and professional. It takes an extensive amount of work to study the health connection between the gut and the brain, but this topic is of importance for parents to help their kids thrive and live productive lives.

By purchasing this book, you will have gained a sense of deep understanding of a subject that has only been theorized between research scientists and experts in their field. You'll have a better perception of the underlying psychology of your child and will become an exceptional parent that can remedy their health needs.

As guardians of our loved ones, we have a responsibility to protect our children and step forward into our caretaking role when the authorities we trust fail to do so. It's up to us to become well informed for our families well being and this book will be your guide for practical yet extensive research on this topic.

You're going to gain a comprehensive understanding of the foods that are negatively affecting the health of your household, as well as the correct ones that should be a part of any diet. The link between mental health and regulation of our moods will become clear as you see their cause-and-effect relationship in the body.

With a better knowledge of nutritional information at hand, you'll better prepare healthy meals for your home and will be well aware of the types of foods you're purchasing on a regular basis. What you may have learned about dieting and healthy eating has been somewhat disingenuous for the most part, as the latest research has disclosed what scientists have been uninformed about for many years.

In our digital world of technology and social media, you're besieged with a vast amount of information everyday. Legitimate knowledge about taking care of your health is lost in the midst of click-bait and popular fad articles that mislead their target audience. This book will expand your mind with a true understanding of the importance of managing your health and taking responsibility for the well being of your kids.

Shea McCrae

ONE

The Brain-Gut Connection

I t's said that 75% of your immune system is in the stomach and yet 70 million report digestive issues in the US alone. It's important to emphasize not only gut health but its impact on the brain as the most crucial aspect of it. Your digestive tract is directly connected to the brain and plays a central role in relaying communication signals in the body.

Your gastrointestinal tract is the part of the digestive system that is responsible for the delivery of the food that enters your mouth to the nutrients that are broken down in the stomach. Absorption of these nutrients occur in the small and large intestines, where waste matter is disposed of from the body. The enzymes and acids that are located in the stomach are tasked with this breakdown of food particles into smaller matter. The microscopic bacteria, better known as the microbiome, line the walls of the stomach and co-exist to further assist the digestion of the food molecules.

The microbiome is composed of a variety of organisms, from bacteria, viruses, and fungi. These organisms form a harmonious relationship with each other and assist the operations of the stomach. Gut health is a phrase that describes the diversity and balance of this microbiome. When either of these organisms are imbalanced, we can encounter noticeable health symptoms that can later become problematic.

Each species of bacteria has a different function in the body and some counters the actions of others. Some bacteria can activate immune cells while others can turn them off. Other bacteria can release particles that cause inflammation, and bacterial organisms with anti-inflammation properties can also co-exist in the same environment.

This is why gut health becomes important, as these imbalances cause susceptibility to sickness and allergies. Signs of poor gut health include bloating, gas, diarrhea, stomach pain, nausea, weight loss, constipation, sudden weight loss, jaundice, and trouble swallowing food. If you recognize any of these symptoms after any of your meals this could be of concern. Further studies of these imbalances in humans have also found a connection to chronic conditions such as type II diabetes, cancer, heart disease, and multiple sclerosis.

Because of how the gut is connected to the nervous system, these imbalances affect how we feel mentally. When we feel nervous or anxious, this causes hormones to be released that change the compositions of our microbiome. This is why someone that is preparing to speak in public or perform on stage may observe that they're 'feeling butterflies in their stomach' right before the event. Mental stress has a tendency to cause an upset stomach and even change your appetite.

Stress is able to make such an impact on the stomach because of the receptors lining the entire GI tract known as the ENS. The ENS, or enteric nervous system, are 100 million nerve cells that regulate the release of enzymes in the stomach, distinguish nutrients or waste products, and even control the mechanism of swallowing. These sensory neurons embedded in the digestive tract stretch from the lower third of the esophagus to the rectum.

This gut lining of the stomach becomes more permeable whenever we encounter stress. When stressor signals are delivered throughout the body, content from inside the gut leaks into the bloodstream without being properly filtered from bad microbes. This transmission of unhealthy organisms out of the gut is known as 'leaky gut' and can have a negative impact on an individual's health.

Stress also has the ability to change how the food that is consumed is metabolized in the body and causes changes to the metabolic changes. Studies have shown that those who are under stress may have lower oxidation of fats in the body, increased levels of insulin, and a decreased energy expenditure after consuming a fatty meal.

The gut's functional physiology can also be altered by stress when we encounter stress for prolonged periods of time. Development of conditions such as ulcers or Crohn's disease have been linked back to earlier periods of stress that can date back to early childhood. When impacted with stress, the body's ability to heal itself is reduced and the pH of the gut can become less acidic, which causes indigestion, heartburn, reflux, and other problems.

Whenever you get into a stressful situation, a flight or fight response is stimulated, which releases a hormone called *cortisol* that keeps your body on high alert. The high alert status can change the pH of the stomach, leading to bloating or feeling nauseous. The ENS becomes overstimulated and the esophagus can go into spasms.

This is a breakthrough for modern science, as research has discovered that overstimulation of the ENS may be a cause behind anxiety, depression, and common problems of the bowels. Previous studies indicated that the anxiety and depression was creating problems in the GI tract, which left many patients feeling helpless about their gut issues. Having a clear understanding of this cause and effect relationship with the ENS empowers individuals to take a steadfast approach in resolve to their gut health.

This new information brings light to a treatment that can involve the ENS connection with the central nervous system, or the CNS. Mind-body therapies such as cognitive brain therapy and medical hypnotherapy resolves GI issues by getting the nervous system between the gut and the brain to communicate with each other effectively. In the near future we should have a clearer understanding of how these systems relay signals in response to the variety of nutrients present in our diets.

The connection between this brain-gut axis is made possible by the vagus nerve, which is like the main highway in the network of nerves that transports messages in both directions routinely. Whenever we experience stressors from our environment, this stops the flow of this highway and causes disruptions in the transmission of these signals. People who experienced IBS or Crohn's disease were found to have reduced vagal nerve tone, indicating this nerve pathway was damaged.

Signals that establish communication between the brain and the gut are chemicals known as neurotransmitters. Neurotransmitters are released from their source and are sent to the targeted cellular membrane through receptors. Neurotransmitters are also responsible for maintaining homeostasis, or overall balance in the human body.

Neurophine, epinephrine, dopamine, and serotonin are able to regulate and control blood flow, affect gut motility, nutrient absorption, the gut's innate immune system, and the microbiome. Serotonin plays a specific role of moderating gastric secretion and body temperature control. Dysfunctional serotonin levels in the stomach can impair brain functions such as mood, sleep, and behavior.

The precursor to serotonin is tryptophan, which is an essential amino acid found in meat, dairy, and fruits. Once tryptophan is processed, it enters the blood-brain barrier and is later converted to serotonin in the brain stem. The gut microbiome regulates the metabolic pathway for tryptophan, which will influence the conversion of serotonin that's affecting brain cognition and digestive tract function. Less than 1% of available tryptophan is converted to serotonin and this amount is broken down by two enzymes that compete for this amino acid. Serotonin dysfunction can also result from tryptophan levels being depleted.

Since the gut is in direct communication with your brain, the microbiome plays a big part in the compounds that will affect your physical and mental health. Specific types of bacteria in the gut produce short chain fatty acids, known as SCFAs, when they ingest fiber from the foods you consume. These SCFAs have a direct effect on our brain as they're what form the blood-brain barrier and have an impact on lowering appetite. This is why eating fiber rich foods tend to give us feelings of satiety longer than foods without them.

For this reason, it's much easier to transform the gut than discovering new therapies to treat the brain. Scientists have been making the connection between chronic ailments such as Alzheimer's and Parkinsons' disease with new findings that are changing research throughout the world. These diseases of the nervous system seem to have a causative factor in common: inflammation.

In general, when an area of the body is referred to as 'inflamed', it's commonly associated with pain and swelling from an injury or trauma. Inflammation is the immune system's response to a stimulus that is foreign or toxic to your body, which can include antigens. These antigens are the proteins on the surface of bacteria, viruses, fungi, or foreign particles that cause the response from the body.

When there's an inflammatory response without the presence of any foreign invader, it's likely a result from an imbalanced gut microbiome. Without the presence of an invader to remove from the body, the immune system proceeds to attack healthy tissue, which is where the pain and swelling begins to develop. If you never find the underlying issue that caused the inflammation in the first place, this is what leads to chronic issues that manifest into diseases further on.

The modern diet has been linked to the source of many of these inflammatory responses within the body, as most Western diets consist of refined carbohydrates, refined grains, and processed foods. It's been shown that these foods affect your gut microbiome by feeding bacteria that produce inflammatory proteins and leak out of the gut into the bloodstream. This leaky gut condition is where health problems are created elsewhere in the body, as we see with Parkinsons' and Alzheimer's illnesses.

There has been hesitancy from researchers to isolate Parkinsons' disease to bacteria that may have invaded or had overgrowth in the gut, however the studying of Parkinsons' patients has observed recurring conditions of constipation. As mentioned earlier, constipation is one of the symptoms resulting from the ENS being overstimulated, which can affect the entire GI tract. As the ENS and CNS are in direct communication with each other through a common pathway, it's being researched whether these inflammatory stressors could travel to the brain and cause the tremor response seen in Parkinsons' patients.

Inflammation is usually connected to a dysfunctional gut microbiome and can also include oral and dental disorders, hypersalivation, difficulty swallowing, gastro-paresis (delayed digestion), and defecatory dysfunction. These underlying symptoms cause difficulty in treating Parkinson's patients, as the medication to relieve body tremors is not properly absorbed and alternative methods for drug delivery have to be used. These conditions show the gut could be the starting part for pathology of Parkinson's and is integral to treat gut dysbiosis, or gut imbalance, before administration with pharmaceutical drugs.

Inflammatory markers have been associated with Alzheimer's as well, as this condition results from a deterio-ration of the brain's neuron cells. When patients with cases of mild to severe dementia were examined for their levels of bile in the stomach, results showed the individuals with severe dementia had the lowest levels of bile than patients with mild cases. High bile levels are indicators of the pres-ence of good bacteria populations in the gut, as these bacteria produce extra bile as an anti-pathogenic response against bad bacteria. When bile levels are low, bad bacteria have an opportunity to multiply and create problems in other areas of the GI tract.

As with Parkinson's, inflammation is a major contrib-utor to the progression of Alzheimer's, because of immune responses in the brain that impair synapses and neuron cells. It's the degeneration of these vital cells that can lead to the build up of tau protein that creates plaquing between the neurons. This build up can be healthy, as there are both 'good' tau and 'bad' tau protein. When tau proteins are functioning normally, a protein within the neuron known as the amyloid-beta is expelled outside the cell and forms plaque. If tau protein is dysfunctional, this amyloid-beta protein builds up inside the cell and kills the neuron.

Tau protein modification to 'bad' protein can occur much sooner than plaquing in the brain, which is closely connected to diagnosis of early onset dementia. Patients with scans of plaquing in the brain are not always correlated with dementia or Alzheimer's. It's theorized that the gut biome plays a major role in the process of this tau modification, which can be a major risk factor for contracting the disease. Other risk factors for tau modification leading to Alzheimer's are type 2 diabetes, obesity, brain injury, cerebrovascular disease, and hypertension.

By now you should have an idea of how gut health has an impact on your physical function, psychological well being, and the possible outcomes of neglecting it over time. The biochemical processes that occur in our bodies are relatively new knowledge for science but our understanding of the proper nutrients to feed ourselves have been here for generations.

Several reactions occur when food enters our digestive system and is broken down within the gut. Neurotransmitters produced in the stomach that elevate mood and increase cognition are released based on the types of foods consumed in your diet. Foods that are not easily digested benefit the microbes living in the gut, which create proteins that aid and support the health of the brain. A poor diet creates more dysfunction in the digestive tract and the microbes send signals indicating that there is an imbalance.

Modern diets don't give any justice to healthy, strong, and well functioning bodies in the long term. Now with knowledge of what your gut does for your health, we'll move on to more practical advice in Chapter 2.

. . .

CHAPTER SUMMARY

The gut microbiome is composed of a variety of organisms; bacteria, viruses, and fungi that all form a harmonious relationship together and assist in the functions of the stomach. The connection between the brain-gut axis is made possible by the vagus nerve, which transports messages in both directions routinely. Since the gut is in direct communication with your brain, the microbiome plays a big part in the compounds that will affect your physical and mental health. The modern diet has been linked to the source of many inflammatory responses within the body because most Western diets consist of refined carbohydrates, refined grains, and processed foods. This creates chronic inflammation and inflammatory markers have been associated with Alzheimers. The diagnosis of Alzheimers is a condition resulting from a deterioration of the brain's neuron cells.

In the next chapter you will learn about the body's immune system and its relationship with the gut...

TWO

Getting Off on the Right Foot

As Heather Morgan said: "Everytime you eat or drink, you're either feeding disease or fighting it." Knowing if you are doing one or the other is a great start to our journey. This philosophy often comes second nature to those that receive urgent information from a physician that their health is at risk, but what about those who recognize there is more to eating than suspending hunger until the next meal? It would be wise to consume the right foods that aid and build our gut health to avoid the disastrous outcome of a poor diet. When you support the body's organ health, it reciprocates that effort and supports you back.

The Immune System

The body's defense system helps us the most when we're the most vulnerable and dependent on it. The immune system functions like a meticulous bookkeeper, keeping track of every microbe that enters the body, assembling the appropriate arsenal, and eliminating it when detected in the future. When the immune system is working optimally, it responds to a potential threat that could damage the tissues or organs in its proximity in a timely manner. What you experience as symptoms from illness or an infection is your immune system doing what it does best. Healthy individuals—people with strong immune systems— are expected to have quick recoveries.

The immune system is composed of the white blood cells, the antibodies, the complement system, the lymphatic system, the spleen, the thymus, and the bone marrow.

White blood cells originate in the bone marrow and circulate through the blood system searching for foreign organisms to be eliminated if identified. White blood cells have varieties ranging from B-Cells, T-Cells, and natural killer cells that each have specific roles in the defense system.

Antibodies help eliminate organisms by marking the antigens on the microbe for destruction. Once the organism has been marked, an assortment of chemicals, proteins, and cells are used to eliminate the pathogen. The proteins that work with these antibodies are known as the complement system.

The lymphatic system is a circulatory pathway that regulates cellular waste products, body fluid levels, fatty acids in the bloodstream, and dispurses healthy white blood cells to the appropriate areas in the body. Fluids leaking from the body's tissues are drained by the lymphatic system back into the circulating blood. If fluids are not drained, this can result in edema, or swelling in the body. The lymphatic system also absorbs fats, fat soluble vitamins, and proteins from your intestines and transports them into the bloodstream.

To filter toxins from the body, the lymphatic system uses round nodules located in the neck, armpits to store viruses, bacteria, and fungi for later elimination. They also produce and store additional white blood cells to be transported throughout lymph vessels throughout the body. Smaller lymph vessels known as lymph capillaries drain fluids away from the tissues into the larger vessels. One of these main vessels are the thoracic duct that drains from the lower spine, pelvis, abdomen, and lower chest. The other is the right lymphatic duct that collects lymph from the right side of the neck, chest, and arm.

The spleen is an organ that repairs damaged red blood cells and clears microbes from circulating blood. It's part of the lymphatic system, which is also a part of your immune system. The spleen is also responsible for making substances that's important for inflammation and healing. There are two parts of the spleen; the white pulp and red pulp. The white pulp is responsible for producing white blood cells that create antibodies for infections. Red pulp acts as a filter, removing waste and getting rid of old or damaged red blood cells. This red pulp also fights viruses and bacteria.

The other filtering organ is the thymus, which also produces white blood cells. This gland is the training ground for white blood cells to develop, grow, and select T lymphocytes to fight infections and foreign invaders. The thymus also releases a hormone that induces an immunological effect, where the lymphocyte cells that are affected can recognize pathogens and invaders accurately. Humans are born with a full complement of T cells in circulation and lymphoid tissue, with the thymus being the largest at birth up until puberty. When an individual reaches the age of an adult, this gland begins to shrink and is gradually replaced by fatty tissue.

Bone marrow is the porous tissue located in the interior of the skeletal bones. This tissue creates red blood cells for carrying oxygen, white blood cells for fighting foreign organisms, and platelets that clot the blood. There are two types of bone marrow that fills the inside of your bones: red bone marrow and yellow bone marrow.

Red bone marrow hosts stem cells that can develop into different types of cells: red blood cells, platelets, and white blood cells. As you age this bone marrow is eventually replaced by yellow bone marrow. This bone marrow can only be found in the skull, vertebrae, sternum, ends of the upper arm, pelvis, ends of the thigh bone, and ends of the shin bone.

Yellow bone marrow is involved in the storage of fats. The fats are stored in cells known as adipocytes that can be accessed for the release of energy when needed. Yellow marrow also contains mesenchymal stem cells that can develop into muscle, fat, bone, or cartilage tissue.

Like other organ systems, the immune system has disorders that cause it to not function well. When the system overreacts, a harmless substance like pollen or dust particles could activate antibodies to attack this allergen. Allergic reactions are some of the most common health conditions in the world population. They can include allergies to foods, medications, insect bites, anaphylaxis, hay fever, sinus disease, asthma, hives, dermatitis, and eczema.

When normally functioning organs are attacked from within the body, this can create chronic ailments that later need treatment. Autoimmune disease is a term to describe more than 100 disorders that can occur. The most recognized mechanisms behind autoimmunity disorders are excessive hygiene, cellular mimicry, and intestinal leaky gut. These lead into the main triggers for disorder, which are food, chemical exposures, infections and microbiome imbalances, nutritional deficiencies, and chronic stress levels. The list of diseases include multiple sclerosis, rheumatoid arthritis, type 1 diabetes, Hashimoto's thyroid disease, Crohn's disease, ulcerative colitis, and many others. Autoimmune disorders can affect many different tissues and organs in the body, causing a variety of symptoms including pain, fatigue, drowsiness, nausea, headaches, dizziness, and more.

With an underactive immune system, the body is unable to defend itself from viruses, bacteria, and parasites. Having a weaker immune system that is susceptible to infection is also known as immunodeficiency, which can be temporary or permanent. If you're born with a deficiency disease, it's called a primary immunodeficiency disorder. Common primary immunodeficiency disorders include common variable immunodeficiency (CVID), severe combined immunodeficiency (SCID), and chronic granulomatous disease (CGD).

Immunity diseases that have occured from an outside source is known as a secondary immunodeficiency disorder. Severe burns, chemotherapy, radiation, diabetes, and malnutrition are all contributing factors that can lead to this condition. Examples of secondary immunodeficiency disorders are AIDS, leukemia, viral hepatitis, multiple myeloma are diseases that lowers immunity from a reduction of healthy white blood cells circulating in the blood.

Immune system vitality is also lowered through the administration of chemical treatments, such as with corticosteroids and chemotherapy. Chemical therapies are often used as a precursor to prevent the occurrence of autoimmune diseases and other ailments. For example, corticosteroids were designed to suppress the immune system by making the white blood cells inactive and reduce the likelihood for inflammation. Chemotherapy is another immunosuppressant that destroys cancer cells and inadvertently kills healthy white blood cells, causing the remaining immunity cells to not work properly. This can leave you vulnerable to infections.

GUT-IMMUNE SYSTEM RELATIONSHIP

The immune system has a strong affinity with the bacteria that lives in the gut, which encompasses the microbiota. The gut microbiota is composed of 100 trillion organisms that live in the gastrointestinal tract, sharing a mutually beneficial relationship with the body's cells. These organisms impact nearly every major function within our body, including memory and cognitive performance, weight management, mood, and digestion.

The microbiota works with this immune system to make sure these functions of the body are working optimally at all times. This begins when the body is introduced to a large amount of bacteria from the birth canal, where the immune system can learn and develop its strength. To prevent the white blood cells from attacking the body's own cells, the microbiome teaches the immune cells to distinguish the human cells from foreign pathogens. When this is accomplished, the gut biome sends signals for healthy immune response in exchange for more health-promoting microbes.

It's crucially important that there is an established communication between the gut microbiota and immune system to prevent any disorders or diseases from occurring. Gut microbes play key roles with inflammatory signaling by interacting directly and indirectly with immunity cells. Some bacteria ferment complex carbohydrates to create short chain fatty acids that modulate immune cells. Short chain fatty acids (SCFA) are one of the most abundant byproducts of microbes in the gut and have the ability to reduce intestinal inflammation, protect against pathogen invasion, and maintain gut lining integrity.

These SCFAs are also crucial for the activation, recruitment, and differentiation of immune cells, including neutrophils, macrophages, and T lymphocytes. One of the SCFAs, butyrate, is essential in suppressing inflammatory responses in the body and has a strong presence in the makeup of the blood/brain barrier. Butyrate also changes the pH of the gut to create an inhospitable environment for pathogens to proliferate and colonize the microbiome.

Every individual's gut microbiota is dynamic and changes depending on age, geographic location, diet, antibiotic use, physical damage to the mucus lining, and influx of microbes from their environment. Gut dysbiosis refers to the mutation of the microbiota that have harmful effects on the host's health by changes in the quantity of microbes, difference in microbe activity, or the redistribution of microbes along the digestive tract. Friendly bacteria not only change the environment conditions, but they also change the expression of the pathogen's genes.

If good microbes are removed by poor lifestyle choices or inducing toxins into your body with chemicals, this creates an imbalance in gut health and weakens the strong relationship with the immune system. Human gut dysbiosis has a close relationship with diseases. Gut dysbiosis causes immune dysregulation and increases the risks of developing conditions such as inflammatory bowel syndrome (IBS), diabetes, obesity, cardiovascular disease, infectious diseases, and autoimmune disease. The good news is that imbalances can be reversed by consuming probiotic foods that promote the population of healthy microbes, such as sauerkraut, kefir, and specific types of yogurts or dairy.

· · ·

GUT HEALTH **and Behavior**

Gut microbes are also part of the unconscious system that regulates behavior. As humans are naturally social creatures and microbiota had a co-evolutionary past together, social engagement was a benefit for development of our brains and the natural exchange of healthy microbes within our species. In fact, the microbes acquired during your lifetime plays a part in the development of personality and social interaction.

The composition of our microbiota could make a difference in our social behavior from the pathways of the gut/brain axis. A study conducted with mice that were raised without a microbiome and administered indigenous bacteria, the subjects were observed to prefer engaging social interaction with other mice instead of a novel object. Analysis of the amygdala region of the brain that controls social behavior showed an increase of brain derived neurotrophic factor from the presence of these microbes.

When we have deficiencies in this social interaction and lack abilities to communicate properly, this condition is known as autism spectrum disorder (ASD). Fetuses that introduce their microbiota to bacteria from the birth canal, also known as maternal immune activation, have differing levels of social interaction to fetuses birthed through cesarean operational procedures. In an experiment conducted with mice that were diagnosed with ASD behavior pathways, administering probiotics corrected behavior abnormalities, treated communicative defects, and cured gut permeability.

In addition, stress plays a role in the response and behavior traits of those with a compromised microbiome. Environmental stressors can cause a torrent of flight or fight response hormones to be released into the blood-stream, which usually results in anxious or erratic behavior patterns. As with mice in the ASD experiment, probiotics delayed the response of cortisol and adrenocorticotropic hormone (ATCH) during stress restraints. When the body is in a condition of stress, the region of the brain that scans your environment for danger known as the amygdala adapts behavior patterns for the body's safety and survival.

Maternal separation is another stressor that can dramatically change behavior and the diversity of the microbiota. For treatment of these emotional processes psychobiotics are administered that have effects to positively alter behavior patterns. These bacteria are capable of releasing gamma-aminobutyric acid and serotonin, which are neurotransmitters that have positive effects on your mood. 90% of this serotonin is produced in the gut and a majority of the cell receptors are located there as well.

The anti-inflammatory actions of these psychobiotics could be responsible for alleviating conditions of depression, chronic fatigue syndrome, and irritable bowel syndrome (IBS). Resilience to environmental stressors would otherwise be treated with medication that controls only the flawed behavior and not the root of the problem, which is the imbalance microbiota. Research from a study in 2015 had shown that 50% of patients recovered with the administration of psychiatric medication, while the other 50% who were still experiencing symptoms are struggling with issues from mental health. These individuals may have the side effects of the medication but without relief of the symptoms. If we can learn to manipulate the gut microbiome through the power of psychobiotics to impact mental well being, this can be a super powerful goal and outcome in nutritional psychiatry.

. . .

TESTING KIDS' **Gut Health**

When you see something is not right or hear a complaint from any of your children, the first response is to get a professional evaluation as a confirmation. It would almost seem negligent to not do so and if you're not timely the situation could get much worse.

The same discretion is applicable when it comes to being proactive concerning your kids' gut health. Testing how well the flora in the digestive tract is working will mainly rely on observing the quality of excrement and frequency of visits to the bathroom. You do have several options in going about this, so I'll take you through a step by step itinerary that you can follow:

1. This one will be the simplest of any of the testing protocols, which is a standard visual test. When you investigate this you want to check for two things: visual color and physical indicators.

2. Generally speaking, the color of stool signifies how well the food is being digested properly in the tract. Green color is the least to worry about, as this indicates that the vegetables in the diet aren't being digested enough. Yellow stool is a sign of inflammation in the GI tract and should be addressed when possible. Black and red stool is of the greatest concern as this signals internal bleeding, unless you've fed your child beets in any of their meals (more on this later).

3. The physical indicators of your child's stool will have to also be taken account of as this can vary greatly. The consistency of their excrement will vary from signs of constipation or diarrhea based on the Bristol Stool Chart,

which you can look up anywhere online to analyze further. If you observe signs of either constipation or diarrhea this should be noted with the other indicators.

4. Stools that float or sink are indicators of the content of their bowel movements; floating means there is a high presence of fatty acids and sinking is signs that there are nutrients that are not being digested. Your child's frequency of restroom visits are also signals of either normal gut health.

5. The next test involves using beets to test the speed of digestion. After serving beets at one of their meals, wait 24-48 hours to observe a change in color of the stool to a reddish/black color. This one may be the most challenging as most kids aren't keen on eating a lot of vegetables, much less one's we try to force on them! The beets only have to be one serving at one meal, so it shouldn't be too much to ask.

6. If you want to get a full professional view of what may be going on regarding gut health, a functional stool test is highly recommended. A stool sample is sent to a lab for inspection and a printout report is sent back displaying various information about the microbiome. Bacteria overgrowths, enzyme levels, nutrient malabsorption, and strains of microflora are some of the data you'll receive back once the test is completed. To get one done you'll need to work with a functional medicine doctor where a test can be conducted from the office. These tests are quite expensive to evaluate but

may be worth it to get a definitive analysis on any issues that need your attention.

7. If any of your kids are suffering from bloating or a condition of SIBO (small intestinal bacterial overgrowth) then you should request a lactulose breath test. This test is conducted over 24 hours with a modified diet, consuming a sugary beverage, and periodically testing their breath for SIBO conditions.

Our kids' gut health is intertwined with so many of the body's functions that affect their quality of life. The gut acts as a gauge of how well you're taking care of your health with the choices you make with your lifestyle.

The immunity, mental health, and hormonal pathways are all impacted by the gut, so you should test your kids occasionally to see how well they're doing. Simple observations that could be done at the house are accurate for the most part. If food is not passing through the digestive tract properly, stool tests will determine if there are any issues. Functional testing may be necessary if the quality of excrement has not changed after a lengthy period of time or conditions are getting worse. A professional evaluation could give you a second opinion on refinements needed to be made in the diet for progress.

Most of the symptoms of poor gut health are reversible, however, these conditions can become quite serious when you're not proactive enough. Most illnesses are the result of not understanding their true natural causes and the measures that would prevent them. Moving on to Chapter 3, we cover some of the changes one has to make in search of these improvements to aid their gut health optimally.

. . .

CHAPTER SUMMARY

When the immune system is optimal, it responds to a potential threat that could damage the tissues or organs in a timely manner. The immune system can then become dysfunctional, such as with an overreaction to an allergen or autoimmune responses in the body. Examples of these diseases are multiple sclerosis, rheumatoid arthritis, type 1 diabetes, and Hashimoto's. The immune system has a strong affinity with the microbiota, which encompasses 100 trillion organisms that live in the digestive tract. It's crucially important that there is an established communication between the gut microbiota and immune system to prevent any diseases or illnesses from occurring.

Fetuses introduce bacteria into their microbiome from passage within the birth canal, better known as maternal immune activation, which helps develop personality and social interaction. The dysbiosis of this healthy gut flora can occur from choices in diet, environmental factors, or the use of antibiotics to treat symptoms related to illness. This imbalance of the microbiome can cause observable mental and behavioral changes in kids suffering from an overgrowth of bad microbes. Get a professional evaluation when observing odd behavior or hearing a complaint from your children to be more proactive. This involves testing how well the fluora in the digestive tract is working and will rely on observing the quality of excrement and frequency of visits to the bathroom. The gut acts as a gauge of your health and the lifestyle choice that works for or against your favor.

In the next chapter you will learn about the foods you need to avoid to have a healthy lifestyle…

THREE

Changes That Might Prove Difficult

S ugar and fat will generally trigger pleasure centers in our brain and this is one of the biggest traps the human body can fall into. We want more in search of energy but this is only a short-term reward. Food has become a source of sedation and escapism since it's readily available for a majority of developed countries throughout the world. Rather than eating for survival, we overindulge in our guilty pleasures until it starts to become an obstacle in our lives.

To bring balance back into our lives, we have to make adjustments to the sources of food that's preventing us from having the quality of health that we truly deserve. Getting rid of the junk that's bad for you AND the foods you may not have been aware of is what's necessary to improve health. In addition we need to add substances that are deficient from most standard diets for a variety of reasons. These improvements can be applied for those that are the most resistant to change, as the satisfying results from change are always guaranteed in the long term.

. . .

WHAT YOU WILL NEED **to Abandon**

Most of the foods that our kids' enjoy have been advertised and marketed to them for many years. Kids tend to crave foods they're familiar with that are not the healthiest options while being very hesitant trying nutrient dense, natural whole foods. It would be ideal to feed kids these healthy foods, however many parents are unaware that these 'natural' whole foods contain harmful contaminants and toxic compounds. If we have a better understanding of the sources of these toxins and what they're doing to our bodies, we can take further steps in the right direction in regards to our nutrition.

NATURAL TOXINS

Some plants that exist in nature have defense mechanisms to protect themselves from predators, insects, and microorganisms when threatened. These chemicals that are released are known as natural toxins that are harmless for the plants but are toxic when consumed by humans or other species. Many of the common foods that we enjoy have small amounts of these toxins within them, but these poisons can affect our health negatively when consumed in high doses. Vegetables and certain fruits can also contain what's known as lectins that cause irritation within the gut for some individuals, even when consumed in small amounts. Some of these foods include tomatoes, cucumbers, all legumes, soy based products, and peas. These symptoms include diarrhea, vomiting, lightheadedness, nausea, stomach pains, dizziness, paralysis, neurological issues, coma, and even death. The best way to avoid intoxication is to physically check your food for signs of mold, bruising, discoloration, or foul odors that could be emitting from it. Eating any foods from the wild, especially mushrooms, should be done with precaution. Throw the food away if the plant has an unusual taste or does not taste particularly fresh.

ARTIFICIAL INGREDIENTS

Additives are usually included to preserve shelf life, improve flavor, or make the appearance of food more appealing. Of course, these lab made products are all artificial ingredients and are present in many foods in most grocery aisles. This is a list of the most common ones and the food where they're found often.

Monosodium Glutamate

Monosodium Glutamate (MSG) is a flavor enhancer that has the properties of salt and protein. It changes the taste profile of many foods that would be otherwise bland and tasteless, which is why it's often found in packaged foods, microwave meals, salty snacks, and canned soups. Often manufacturers will have their labels display 'No MSG' on the packaging, when the MSG ingredient has been hidden as 'hydrogenated proteins' or 'autolyzed yeast extract'. Manufacturers will try to hide disclosure of this ingredient as MSG has been known to cause change in blood glucose levels, which can be problematic for individuals suffering from metabolic syndrome (heart conditions, obesity, blood pressure, etc.)

Artificial Colors

Artificial food color is one of the additives used to decorate the appearance of foods to make them more attractive to consumers. The main ones used (Red 40, Blue 1, Yellow 5 and 6) have been linked to allergic reactions and hyperactivity, especially with children that are susceptible. These chemicals are toxins because they're derived from petroleum products, which gives them longer shelf life and lower costs than similar natural colors. They provide no nutritional value and may cause irritation and emotional disruption in kids. International food manufacturers have been regulated by Europe and British regulations in those markets; however, artificial food colors continue to be used in products sold in the United States, where similar regulations are not currently in place.

Each dye can affect children differently: red #40 can cause hyperactivity, migraines, impulsiveness, fidgeting, and brain buzzing; green #3 can cause symptoms similar to bipolar disorder; blue #1 can cause irritability moodiness, and fatigue; and yellow #5 & 6 can cause anxiety, aggravation, aggression, defiance, violent outburst, and suicidal thoughts. Artificial colors are often found in beverages (sports drinks), dairy products, candies, confectionery, dry mixes, pie filling, and puddings. Most medications for behavior problems contain artificial food dyes. These coloring additives are associated with health problems such as ADHD, eczema, cancer, confusion, violent outbursts, sleep disturbances, itchiness, and frustration.

To identify products in your home with artificial dyes, look at your ingredients list. As you run out of products that contain dyes, replace them with products that may have natural dyes or none at all. Food dye intolerance can be tested for 2 weeks within children by eliminating the source of these dyes from the diet.

Sodium Nitrates

To extend shelf life and make packaged meat products more profitable in supermarket aisles, sodium nitrate is often used to entice customers. This additive changes the appearance by giving the meat a deep reddish-pink color, which is much more marketable than the true appearance of naturally cured meat. Nitrates can become problematic when they're exposed to high heat or protein, which can turn into nitrosamine. Nitrosamine is known as a carcinogen that is associated with stomach and colon cancer. Nitrosamine also impairs motor function and learning degeneration of the nervous system. Also nitrates can increase the risks of type 1 diabetes, especially in kids. Nitrates also impair oxygen transport. Foods that you should avoid that have high nitrates contents are ham, hot dogs, bacon, salami, sausages, corned beef, bologna, beef jerky, salted and cured meat, as well as smoked meat. Certain types of vegetables also contain sodium nitrates which can be converted to sodium nitrite in small amounts. They don't pose the same health risk as nitrites found in processed meats. There are packaged meat options you can purchase that are not prepared with sodium nitrates.

Guar Gum

Guar gum is a thickening agent that's used by the food industry to produce salad dressings, soups, ice cream, nut milks, and sauces. These are mostly processed foods, which should be minimized in any healthy diet. The gum is extracted from the guar bean and has a high fiber content, which helps achieve satiety after consumption. This agent is often used as a replacement for gluten in bread products, which help them retain some of the qualities found in these products. Guar gum is also good as a better alternative emulsifier when used in cooking, in comparison to corn starch or modified food starch.

The downside to this additive is that it can cause mild symptoms of bloating, gas, or cramps with some people, especially in large amounts. Guar gum can also cause an inflammatory reaction in people with soy allergies. This emulsifier is also made from a legume, which contains lectins that can be hard to digest and irritate the digestive system. If you use too much guar gum powder, it can soak up all the water in the large intestine and cause constipation. Food additives in general can throw off the bacterial balance in your gut, and that can set the stage for autoimmune disease, intestinal permeability, and inflammation. If any of these symptoms are occuring you may just want to search for products without the agent.

High Fructose Corn Syrup

Sweeteners are known additives that are found in various forms in many of the foods we purchase on store shelves. High fructose corn syrup is a more dangerous additive than sugar due to the composition of this sweetener. It's also toxic because it's made in a lab and is extracted from corn, which is a GMO. There are other chemical contaminants that are used in the manufacturing, such as chloralkali that contains mercury that's found in beverages and many other products that use high fructose corn syrup. Currently the average American is consuming about 34 grams of high fructose per day. Theoretically if you were getting the most contaminated corn syrup, you could exceed your mercury limits by consuming the average amount of corn syrup without eating any other mercury containing food.. This source of sugar has also been treated with glyphosate from RoundUp ready corn that has been harvested.

While sucrose has a 50/50 ratio of glucose to fructose that is bound together, high fructose corn syrup ratio is 55/45 and is unbound. This unbound fructose is what creates a lot more liver damage, similar to the effect of drinking alcohol. Fructose is the toxic simple sugar that can only be digested by the liver in the body, which can overtax the organ if large quantities are indigested at once. This is due to a process known as lipogenesis, which is fat production in the liver as a result of excess fructose being digested. Kids have the highest consumption of high fructose corn syrup with over 72 grams per day, which is equivalent to about 60lbs per person each year.

High fructose corn syrup can also contribute to other adverse effects such as inflammation in the cell tissue, hypertension, non-alcoholic fatty liver disease, excess uric acid levels (associated with gout), elevated levels of glycated end products (which are linked with diabetes and aging), cancer, and heart disease. HCFS can also affect mental functioning and performance. This sweetener is typically found in breakfast cereals, snack foods, candy, and soda beverages.

Artificial Sweeteners

Artificial sweeteners are used in diet and sugar-free foods and beverages to keep caloric content low and appeal to consumers that are managing their blood glucose levels. Many of these sweeteners are actually 1-6x sweeter than standard sucrose and can simultaneously retrain your taste buds to require more and more sweetness. Sweeteners commonly used in these products are aspartame (Sweet N' Low & Nutrasweet), sucralose (Splenda), acesulfame potassium, and saccharin (Sweet N' Low).

The origins of these artificial sweeteners are often cloaked in mystery and controversy. For example, saccharin was discovered over 100 years ago by a chemist working with a derivative of coal tar. The product was later banned by the U.S. Department of Agriculture because of its relation with the aforementioned toxin benzoate and its widespread use in sweetened products. The following year the decision for banning was reversed, although it was later linked with bladder cancer for many decades afterwards.

Sucralose is the chemical derivative of sucrose, which is made by adding chlorinating the sucrose molecule to rid the calories from consuming this sugar. This sweetener is often the most recommended for weight reduction and substitution for baking goods. Sucarolosc has been marketed for diabetics for years, but recent studies have shown that it spiked insulin levels in the blood after consumption.

Aspartame, the most widely used sweetener in thousands of products, was discovered by a pharmaceutical drug research scientist that was attempting to formulate a new inhibitor drug for ulcers. When a scientist spilled the formula from his flask and tasted his fingers afterward, aspartame was soon created. Symptoms of this chemical include brain cancer, cardiovascular disease, Alzheimer's, fibromyalgia, seizures, stroke, dementia, intestinal dysbiosis, mood disorders, headaches, and migraines.

These products can also shut down the liver, kidneys, and are an excitotoxin (which over-stimulates brain neurons). This occurs in the brain and as well as in peripheral nerves because these sweeteners in free form are readily absorbent and cross the blood-brain barrier. These nerve cells can become excited to the point of cellular death. An imbalance of all these excitotoxins during critical periods of brain development can result in abnormal function of the brain pathways. This can lead to serious behavior problems such as hyperactivity, aggressiveness, learning disorders, attention deficit disorders, infertility, menstrual issues, and premature puberty.

In relation to gut health, new studies have also found that artificial sweeteners reduced gut bacteria by almost 50%, increased the pH level in the intestines, and contributed to intestinal permeability. When possible they should be avoided at all costs because of what occurs when they're processed in the body. These sweeteners can be found in children's vitamins, mouthwash, toothpaste, cough syrup, gum, zero-calorie water beverages, candy, baked goods, snack foods, prepared meats, cereals, and salad dressings.

Sodium Benzoate

Sodium benzoate is a preservative used in carbonated drinks and acidic foods to maintain product shelf life. Sodium benzoate is used often in beverages because it intensifies the flavor from high fructose corn syrup by increasing the acidity. On the back of the soda bottles or cans you can find sodium benzoate listed as E211. Although it's a food preservative, it can also be found in many cosmetics, pharmaceuticals, dyes, and in industrial settings. The preservative is relatively safe to consume in moderation, however when combined with a vitamin C or ascorbic acid, sodium benzoate breaks down into a carcinogenic compound known as benzene. Benzene is found in the highest amounts in cola products and cole slaw. Some of the most common side effects are headaches, confusion, cancer, decreased appetite, increased thirst, dry mouth, and mood swings.

Trans Fat

Products with moderate fat content in general have bad reputations in general, which is what often confuses consumers. Trans fats are unsaturated fats that undergo a process of preservation called hydrogenation, which stabilizes the fat as a solid or liquid at room temperature. There are four main sources of trans fatty acids in the human diet; industrially produced trans fats from the partial hydrogenation of vegetable oils, trans fats produced during the heating process, trans fats that originate from natural animal sources, and trans fats synthesized for the use in dietary supplements. This hybrid type of fat can be packaged in a wide variety of food products ranging from cooking oils, margarine, microwave popcorn, biscuits, and other processed foods.

Industrial trans fats raise low density lipoproteins (LDL) cholesterol levels and lowers high-density lipoproteins (HDL) cholesterol levels, increasing the risk for chronic heart disease. Foods with trans fats have been linked to chronic inflammation, non alcoholic fatty liver disease (NAFLD), and type II diabetes. In animal models, studies have shown changes in the microbiota when industrial trans fats were consumed. When high and low amounts of hydrogenated soybean oil were administered to mice for 8 weeks, a dysbiosis with an abundance of harmful gut bacteria was detected. One species of this bacteria was noted to increase gut permeability due to the microbes byproduct of hydrogen sulfide, which increases inflammation of the gut lining.

As of recently, the FDA has required manufacturers to disclose the content of trans fat in all labeled foods and has revoked their GRAS (generally regarded as safe) status. Manufacturers have found a loophole around this rule as foods with less than 0.5g of trans fat per serving can still be listed as 0g of trans fat on the label. To avoid these products with trans fat, carefully read the ingredients label on the foods you're purchasing and minimize the purchase of processed packaged foods.

Artificial Flavoring

Foods that would have flavors that are difficult or expensive to replicate are often made with artificial flavorings. Artificial flavorings are lab made chemicals that imitate the natural taste synthetically. These flavorings are also generally found in most processed foods and can be present in a wide variety of food products such as spreads, microwave meals, candies, supplement powders, fruit juices, and soda. These foods can become toxic to our bodies, as it can prohibit cellular division of the red blood cells and damage bone marrow tissue. Regularly consuming foods with artificial flavorings can cause high blood pressure, DNA mutations, obesity, infertility, low testosterone in men, nervous system complications, migraines, allergies, and tumors.

Yeast Extract

Yeast extract is an additive used to enhance flavor similarly to MSG (monosodium glutamate). This extract is used as a replacement in 'No MSG' labeled foods to appear as a natural ingredient. Foods with this additive include soups, sauces, broths, baked goods, dairy products, snack goods, some meats, and canned fish. Some individuals have a sensitivity to this additive and can experience some symptoms of elevated blood pressure, headaches, drowsiness, asthma, numbness, and chest pains.

Sugar

Sugar can be both a gift and a curse for our health, as it's both revered and vilified. Sugar, in the form of glucose, is one of the energy sources that the body uses to fuel the cells within our organ systems. Most of the calories that we consume are metabolized into glucose. Whole foods like fruits and vegetables contain glucose packaged with healthy amounts of fiber. Excess glucose in small amounts is reserved as glycogen for later use when our circulating glucose levels are relatively low. It becomes a problem when the body has more sugar than it needs and has to find places to store it if it can't be broken down for energy.

This is what sugar is notorious for, creating havoc when it can't be disposed of quickly. This results in glucose storage in the cells and fructose spillover into the bloodstream. The sugar gets absorbed from the intestine and goes through the portal circulation straight to the liver. The liver is the only molecule that can metabolize the molecule fructose. The fructose overwhelms the liver's capacity to be able to metabolize it and the liver has no choice but to take the excess and turn it into liver fat. When the liver becomes fatty, this manifests as obesity, non alcoholic fatty liver disease, diabetes, high blood pressure, inflammation, and chronic heart disease.

This rush of sugar also affects the cognition of the brain. When sugar in the blood is elevated, this causes a rush of insulin levels that has an effect on the brain cells. This high amount of insulin blocks the effects of leptin, a hormone that controls our feelings of satiety after consuming meals. By eating more fiber this can result in less carbohydrate being absorbed in the gut and allows the brain to receive the satiety signal from leptin sooner than otherwise.

Over the past century, the Western diet has increased their fructose consumption from 15 grams per day to 75 grams per day or more. Most of the processed foods are laden with sugars in the form of high fructose corn syrup as a way to make the product more palatable. During the processing of these foods, fiber and nutrients are removed in order to ensure a longer shelf life in stores and make them easy to transport. This is why the low fiber content in processed ingredients creates excessive calorie consumption and addictive eating pattern behavior. Sugar of various forms is present in most of our foods, but excess sugar consumption is something that we can manage and control.

Adults and children have problems managing daily sugar intake because there's not always a clear guideline disclosure on food products. The average teaspoons of sugar consumption for males is 24 teaspoons, but this amount should actually be closer to 9 teaspoons or 36g per day. Females should have no more than 6 teaspoons or 24g per day. To stay within these limits, you should avoid adding sweetened beverages to meals. There can be up to 250 different names for sugar on labels, with complex names used to associate them as 'healthier' forms of sugar. Read ingredient labels on the foods you purchase and search for alternative names for sugar such as: brown sugar, corn sweetener, corn syrup, fruit juice concentrates, high fructose corn syrup, honey invert sugar, brown rice syrup, malt sugar, molasses, and syrup sugars ending in "-ose" (dextrose, fructose, glucose, lactose, maltose, or sucrose).

Problem Fats

Fats are an essential macronutrient that's needed in your diet, however, it's vital to discern between fats that are good for you and which should be avoided when possible. The benefit of fat is that it is a major source of energy that helps build cell membranes and the tissue that surrounds the nerves. You also need fat to absorb important fat soluble vitamins like A, D, E, and K. Monounsaturated and polyunsaturated fats provide many other benefits in the body and are essential for your overall function and well-being. Saturated fats are useful for bodily functions as well, but serve their purpose better in limited amounts.

The fats that have a bad reputation are trans fats, that are present in a majority of processed foods on store shelves and restaurants that use hydrogenated cooking oils to prepare their food. Trans fats are the worst kind of fat because they are essentially foreign to the body because of their composition. The trans fats have bonds in their structure that cannot be broken down properly by the body, so it's assimilated into the cellular membrane and tissues. When this happens cell permeability becomes reduced, which contributes to disorders and diseases such as insulin resistance, chronic heart disease, elevated bad cholesterol level, type II diabetes, stroke, Alzheimer's, and neurological issues.

Healthy fats that are good for us originate from natural sources, such as nuts, seeds, fish, and some vegetables. Monounsaturated fats are completely different from saturated and trans fats because there are less hydrogen atoms attached to the carbon chain, which means that these fats always stay liquid at room temperature. The best sources of monounsaturated fats are olive oil, avocado oil, peanut oil, walnut oil, and high oleic sunflower or safflower oil.

Polyunsaturated fats are sourced from the same foods as monounsaturated fats except they differ from the amount of double bonds in their carbon structure. These double bonds offer health benefits in the body and are identified as either omega-3 fatty acids or omega-6 fatty acids. Omega-3s found in salmon, walnuts, mackerel, sardines, and flaxseeds help lower bad cholesterol, lower triglycerides in the blood, reduce rheumatoid arthritis, balance heart rhythms, and rebuild the protective sheath surrounding the neurons and nerve tissue in the body. When consumed with omega-6 fatty acids, they ideally should reach a balanced ratio of 1:1. Western diets tend to have a higher consumption of omega-6 present since seafood is not consumed as regularly as with other regions of the world. Supplementing the diet with these healthy omega-3 would be essential for maintaining a balanced fatty acid profile in the body.

GMO FOODS

Genetically modified organisms (GMOs) are crops that have been biologically altered to influence the resistance to insects and weeds that would otherwise destroy their harvest. The gene from one species is inserted into another species to alter the appearance and the mechanics of what that plant can do. This can extend the crop's shelf life, emit brighter color, or even change the nutrient density. The creator of this technology, Monsanto, intends for these crops to be herbicide ready when sprayed with a product called Round-up.

Proponents of GMO foods vouch that these crops are beneficial to feed the world's population and that it's advantageous for farmers' agriculture practices. They believe that spraying this herbicide allows the crops to have better yield, however this has not been proven to be the case with many farmers that have purchased GMO seeds and agrochemicals. Once cultivated, 95% of the GMO sold is fed to livestock, which are later consumed by humans that purchase these meat products. The carcass of these animals between those that were eating GMO versus non-GMO are completely unalike, as they look and smell completely different. There's a discoloration that happens over a year with the animals that make them appear older and many of these products are rated poorer and cost less.

These modified foods are toxic to the human body as there aren't any long term studies researching the effects of these crops on our health. RoundUp is classified by the World Health Organization as a class 2A carcinogen, meaning it causes cancer in animals, it causes mutations in human DNA, and where it is sprayed in large amounts it can cause cancer to spread in the population. Studies that have been conducted by the FDA and deemed as safe were only observed for 3 months. Health effects from foods laden with herbicide chemicals are often delayed for 18 or more months, as seen with DDT and DES that were used in the public in the 1950s.

When we consume foods that are GMO, the genetic material from the digested matter is not recognized by the gut bacteria. Within most GMOs, they put in a gene that's called an antibiotic resistant gene. If the gene transfers into bacteria and creates antibiotic-resistant pathogenic bacteria, we can lose the effectiveness of our antibiotics. This is further perpetuated by the RoundUp herbicide, which is a patented antibiotic that's sprayed on a wide variety of the foods you may consume. This creates an antibiotic response in the GI tract, similarly to what was mentioned earlier with autoimmune disease and allergic responses in the body. RoundUp also blocks certain metabolic pathways in the body that are used by the gut bacteria to produce the building blocks of serotonin, melatonin, dopamine, causing the likelihood of ADHD disorders.

Physiological changes in the body with gut bacteria and the biochemistry of RoundUp and its active ingredient glyphosate are strongly correlated and are linked to the explosion of autism in young children. In cases when families switch to organic food, which takes out the GMOSs and toxic chemicals, their kids get better. Genetically modified crops also create allergens because the process of inserting this genetic material creates massive collateral damage within the DNA. In RoundUp ready corn, it has proteins called putrescine and cadaverine which create higher levels of allergens. It's possible that these modified products can also physically alter the digestive tract, as with studies that observed rats that consumed GMO potatoes after 10 days.

Endocrine problems were also observed in another study with rats that were fed Roundup ready corn for their lifetime. It turns out that one of the problems that occurred was damage to the pituitary gland, which is the master gland to the body. Researchers noted that 50 percent of the males and 70 percent of the females died prematurely in comparison to 30 and 20 percent in the control group. The whole process of eating genetically engineered foods may be causing serious disruptions of different systems in the body.

The best way to avoid GMO foods is purchasing organic labeled products when possible. Organic foods cannot be modified, which is why the best places to shop for them are at your local farmer's market. Certain crops grown in the United States are exclusively GMO, such as soy, corn, canola, sugar (from sugar beets), papaya (from Hawaii or China), apples, potatoes, eggplant, zucchini, and squash. Processed packaged foods contain the highest amounts of GMOs, as the oils that they use help keep the products stable for long shelf life.

The number one reported improvement both in terms of people directly, in terms of 3,600 people surveyed with hundreds of doctors, showed an improvement of digestive disorders when removing GMO foods from the diet. Foods that support the liver and kidney cellular detoxification are very important to help remove GMO chemicals that may be stored in organ tissues and other parts of your body. Herbs that can support your health with detoxification are milk thistle, turmeric, cayenne pepper, and dandelion.

WHAT YOU'LL NEED **in Your Meal Plan**

Once you understand why certain foods are bad for your health, it becomes easier to create a meal plan that's valuable. You won't feel guilty eating foods that affect you negatively in the long term and you won't crave foods that are known toxins. Learning about the positive outcomes of eating high quality meals will encourage you to maintain a healthy lifestyle.

. . .

ORGANIC FOOD

Foods sold with the 'organic' label on them are free of synthetic herbicides, pesticides, fungicides, fertilizers, antibiotics, food additives, sewage sludge, irradiation, or bioengineered genes. The levels of organic can range from 50 to 100% certified organic and verification is usually indicated on the package labeling. If something is organic, it doesn't mean that they're not using some type of pesticide, rather the pesticide is less toxic. Organic farmers typically use manure as a source of nitrogen, phosphorus, and potassium. Manure also breaks down more slowly than chemical fertilizers in soil, so the nutrients are released more gradually. There could be a noticeable improvement in your body eating organic labeled foods in comparison with conventional foods. Organic foods have more antioxidant compounds, which can greatly decrease the risk of developing cancer.

Antibiotics are not used in organic products, which protects the microbiota and invasion of antibiotic resistant microbes. Organic fruits and vegetables are also likely to have better nutrient profiles than conventional agriculture because of the natural chemicals and fertilizers used. When farmed produce is sprayed with pesticides and herbicides, it dramatically changes the taste of the food, some are more noticeable than others. Heavily pesticide spray foods are known as the 'dirty dozen', which are a list of fruits and vegetables that contain the highest levels of pesticide residues.

Organic livestock and animal products are raised closer to their natural environments and are not fed hormones, antibiotics, or GMO feed. For meat and dairy products to qualify as organic, the animals must be given organic feed.

Cows and ruminant livestock that eat grass have to be able to graze for ⅓ of the year, while pigs and chickens must have the option to go outside. Because the livestock are grazing on feed that's natural to them, they produce healthy amounts of omega-3 fatty acids in comparison to conventional livestock. The animal byproducts have richer nutrient profiles and are likely to lessen allergic reactions with individuals that are susceptible.

Organic produce can be locally sourced by purchasing from farmer's markets in your town or city. Although not all farmers use organic, the ones that do ensure that their crops are sprayed with natural fertilizers and pesticides. This food is almost always fresher since there isn't a time lapse to getting the produce from the farm to your table. Local produce is picked ripe, unlike major chain supermarkets that source their food from distant farms that ship unripened produce to prevent spoilage during transport.

MONOUNSATURATED AND POLYUNSATURATED **Fats**

To absorb the essential vitamins that your body needs on a regular basis, it's important to have fats as a part of your diet. Certain fats should be moderated while it's important to incorporate a blend of both monounsaturated and polyunsaturated fats into your diet. The reason why these unsaturated fats are so important to your diet is because of the omega-3 and omega-6s fatty acids that must be at a balanced ratio. Since the standard diet has plenty of omega-6 fats, omega-3s aids the cardiovascular system and lower cholesterol levels, especially for individuals that have a history with cardiovascular disease.

Monounsaturated and polyunsaturated fats can be found in almost all oils that are liquid at room temperature: olive, avocado, sunflower, safflower, and cod liver oil. One of the ways you can start eating healthier is by slowly replacing these saturated fats with foods containing more unsaturated fats in your meals. This can be done by substituting nuts for processed snack food items like chips, cookies, or pastries. Cooking can be done with healthy high smoke point oils, such as avocado, to saute or stir-fry home cooked foods. Red meat and poultry can still be included in the diet by trimming the fat and removing the skin to keep the saturated fat content lower. To get a healthier profile of mono and polyunsaturated fats, the meats you purchase should be labeled 'grass fed' and 'grass finished'. These cuts of meat are lean, more nutrient dense, and are fed little to no grain that causes disease and metabolic syndrome within the livestock.

FERMENTED FOOD

Microorganisms added to food can be used to change their appearance, taste, texture, or aroma with a process known as fermentation. This process starts with the breakdown of the glucose components in the food into acidic products being created by the live bacteria. Fermented foods can come from whole food sources like nuts, dairy, vegetables, fruits, cereals, fish, eggs, legumes, nuts, or seeds. Fermentation foods benefit the body because they can introduce additional healthy gut bacteria to our microbiota, which helps support a healthy immune system. Fermentation also increases bioavailability and absorption by your body, which makes the nutrients that are broken down more easily accessible to digest everything.

The positive effects of these fermented foods are likely to be experienced by fermenting your own whole foods at home, instead of a pasteurized product that would have destroyed any good bacteria living within it. Some common fermented foods are homemade kimchi or sauerkraut made with cucumber or cabbage respectively. Herbs can also be fermented as well, such as turmeric and ashwagandha can be more beneficial because you get more phytocompounds that have anti-inflammatory, antioxidant, and probiotic boosting benefits.

Probiotics are the bacteria that provide a host of health benefits in the body once they're consumed. Probiotics like to grow and expand in an acidic environment, which is why organic acids like apple cider vinegar work well for proliferating probiotic bacteria. Prebiotics are fibers that our gut bacteria feed upon to produce healthy proteins and other byproducts. These fibers' byproducts are short chain fatty acids that are released into the blood and affect other organs. To be classified as a prebiotic, this food ingredient must be resistant to the acidic pH of the stomach, be able to be fermented by microbiota, and the growth of intestinal bacteria is stimulated by this ingredient which benefits the host's health. Most fruits and vegetables contain prebiotics, which is why there's little need to introduce these supplements to your diet.

FISH

Fish is a high quality source of protein and healthy fat as a food source. It contains many of the vital trace minerals that are needed by the body daily (potassium, zinc, magnesium, iron, and iodine). Fish is also an excellent source of omega-3 fats, eicosapentaenoic acid (EPA) and docosahexaenoic acid (DHA).

These fatty acids aid in brain function, supporting the vision and nervous system of infants during pregnancy. They also lower the risk of developing dementia, Alzheimers, ADHD, and the development of diabetes. The body doesn't produce either of these two fatty acids, so it has to be supplemented from the foods in our diet. EPA and DHA omega-3s are found in the highest amounts in fatty fish such as salmon, trout, sardines, cod, herring, canned mackerel, and oysters.

The downside of incorporating healthy servings of fish into your diet is the contamination by toxic chemicals. Chemicals such as mercury or PCBs (oily toxins that exist in bodies of water) are present in many fish, particularly the largest fish found in various bodies of water. It's recommended that we eat fatty fish with healthy omega-3s no more than 2-3 times per week to minimize exposure to contaminants. Fish such as mahi mahi or canned tuna should not be consumed more than once per week. Large fish should be avoided altogether by pregnant women and small children.

The items on the supermarket and grocery shelves that we think are harmless can deceive even the most health conscious individuals. It's a lot easier to improve a diet when you learn about the potentially harmful substances in foods that don't provide any benefits for your body or anyone else in your family. If you're willing to improve your gut health, substituting some of the foods that have harmful ingredients for healthier foods is a start in the right direction. Manufacturer labels are quite deceiving because you're not given a clear explanation about what's in the packaging, which many people assume is safe to consume. A list of items to avoid brings a lot of clarity to shopping for your household.

This has covered some of the do's and don'ts when creating a meal plan for you and your kids. However, no individual is the same and the elimination diet discussed in Chapter 4 could make all the difference in solving existing gut problems.

. . .

CHAPTER SUMMARY

Many parents are not aware that 'natural' whole foods contain harmful chemicals and toxic compounds. Foods that have additives to their ingredients lists are usually included to preserve shelf life, improve flavor, or make the product more appealing. Most of the calories we metabolize are turned into glucose, but it becomes a problem when the body has more sugar than it needs and has to find places to store it when not broken down for energy. These can turn into fats, which are a major source of energy that can build cell membranes and tissues that surround the nerves.

When we consume products that are GMOs, the genetic material from the digested matter is not recognized by the gut bacteria. Eating these foods can cause nutritional deficiencies and illness due to a higher concentration of pesticides and herbicides in the diet. Switching over from conventional to organic foods could result in a noticeable improvement in your body. Reasons why are because organic livestock and animal products are raised closer to their natural environments and are not fed hormones, antibiotics, or GMO feed.

To absorb the essential vitamins that your body needs on a regular basis, it's important to have fats as a part of your diet. You can start eating healthier by replacing saturated fats with foods containing more unsaturated fats in your meals. Once you understand why certain foods are bad for your health, it becomes easier to create a meal plan that's valuable. Fish are a good source for high quality protein and healthy fat, but certain varieties are contaminated with toxic chemicals.

In the next chapter you will learn about food intolerance concerning kids and how elimination diets work...

―□―

Building a Happier, Healthier Family, One Reader At A Time.

"Knowledge is power. Knowledge shared is power multiplied."
— *Robert Boyce*

Make a difference in the lives of families struggling with gut and mental health issues. If you've found value in 'Gut Health For Kids: A Parents' Guide to Promoting Brain-Gut Health', we urge you to share your thoughts by leaving a review.

Your words can help others understand the importance of this guide and the positive impact it can have on the health and well-being of children. And don't stop there! Share this book with friends and family who have children and encourage them to take control of their child's health. Together, we can spread the word and help families create a happier and healthier future.

By leaving a review of this book on Amazon, you'll help to signpost the pathway to happy, healthy children and parents, showing new readers where they can find the information they're looking for.

Simply by leaving a brief comment about how this book has helped you and what readers can expect to find inside, you'll help more people find the information they need to put themselves in the driving seat of their family's health and education thereof – to steer themselves in the right direction.

Thank you for helping me on my quest to share my journey with others.

I've made it easy for you to do; just follow the link below to find yourself directly on the review page!

FOUR

Elimination Diet and What to Look Out For

Depending on your kid's metabolism, food tolerance, and behavior, you could be forced into employing an elimination diet sooner or later. The reasoning behind it could influence the waiting period before the reintroduction of foods but the process remains the same.

That is the basic purpose of the elimination diet, to have foods that are believed to cause a 'food intolerance' removed for a short period of time and then later reintroduced to identify whether they are culprits for symptoms. The diet is often a lot more effective than clinical tests, which often don't isolate items of food that cause problems.

Symptoms from food intolerance to observe range from flu-like aches and pains to headaches, hives, itching, stomach and bowel irritation, unusual tiredness, or concentration problems. Because symptoms are unique to each individual, it may take several days to notice signals of intolerance to food.

Various chemicals can be found in natural foods known

to cause food intolerances in people as well. Some of these known substances are salicylates, amines, and glutamates. These would also be categorized as natural toxins as they can cause adverse reactions in some people.

Elimination diets have to be structured differently for each individual because the makeup of our genetic sequence is distinct to one another. The variation in your diet will depend on your food cravings, intolerance symptoms, and choice in diet.

Implementing an elimination diet has been shown to provide benefits that could improve overall health when done correctly. Irritable bowel syndrome (IBS) symptoms of bloating, stomach cramps, and gas are reduced within a few weeks. Eosinophilic esophagitis is a dysfunction of the esophagus that can cause choking to occur when consuming dry and dense foods. Elimination diets are capable of reducing inflammation that causes this allergic reaction.

Restricting foods can also improve ADHD symptoms with children, who are often affected by eating artificially colored and flavored food products. The elimination diet can also help improve skin conditions, such as eczema seen in children and adults from inflammatory foods. When trigger foods are removed from the diet symptoms can completely disappear.

Although elimination diets are the best way to isolate food intolerance symptoms, there are serious risks that should be considered. Because the amount of allowed foods on the diet will be limited for at least a few weeks, there's a likelihood of becoming nutrient deficient. A lack of vitamins and minerals in the diet can stunt growth for children's bodies that are going through hormonal changes. They can also suffer from anaphylaxis when foods are reintroduced because they're more sensitive to these foods. It's recommended that children are monitored by medical professionals while partaking in elimination diets to be cautious and avoid any harm.

The first part of the elimination diet is the removal phase, where the suspected foods are restricted from the diet for no longer than 3 weeks. If symptoms persist after this time period then a doctor would be consulted to further diagnose the individual. Common foods that people typically have allergic or inflammatory responses after they are removed: nuts, seeds, soy, corn, dairy, gluten products, eggs, pork, and seafood. Early in the diet some people observe the symptoms getting worse after removing these foods after the first few days. Symptoms may continue for up to two or three weeks, but they should never become severe allergic reactions with throat swelling or rashes.

Following this removal phase is the reintroduction, where the foods you eliminated are brought back into the diet gradually. When introducing the food group back, you want to observe symptoms over the next 2-3 days and keep a record of how you're feeling or what you're experiencing. It's recommended that you eat a small amount on day one, double that amount on day two, and a larger portion on day 3.

Some symptoms to look out for are joint pain, rashes on the skin, bloating, changes in breathing, headaches, trouble sleeping, fatigue, and changes in bowel habits. If any of the symptoms recur after introducing the food, add it to the 'allergic' list in your food diary and completely remove it from your meal plan. After observing the reaction to the food group over the 3 days, the next group would be reintroduced to continue the process until the completion of the diet.

Elimination diets have been shown to be effective with

children struggling with ADHD, as a 64% improvement in symptoms was observed. Compared to children consuming a standard Western diet no significant changes in behavior was noted. Research conducted as recently as the late 70s show children with ADHD had a 30% improvement from hyperactivity by eliminating foods containing artificial food coloring as additives. These studies and even more recent clinical trials suggest that there is a likely chance for treating ADHD with dietary intervention, which can avoid or delay the use of prescription medication for treatment.

WIDELY USED ELIMINATION **Diets**

Different approaches to the elimination diet can be used to help adults and children with a variety of conditions. The basic elimination diet removes milk, eggs, nuts, added sugars, citrus fruits, wheat, alcohol, shellfish, processed meats, soy, beef, and gluten. After a brief reintroduction period the food group is recorded as neutral or negative for reaction to symptoms.

Gluten Free

Gluten free diets are a type of elimination diet where no protein from wheat products are consumed. This includes barley, rye, tritican, oats, and seitan. Gluten products are also found as additives in many salad dressings and sauces. Processed foods like hot dogs, french fries, tortilla chips, and processed meats contain gluten that could trigger symptoms in those that are sensitive.

FODMAP Diet

The FODMAP diet is a regimen designed to help alleviate the effects of irritable bowel syndrome (IBS) and/or small intestinal bacterial overgrowth (SIBO) in the lower digestive tract. FODMAP restricts small-chain carbohydrates that's poorly digested in the small intestine.

Similarly to the basic elimination diet protocol, FODMAP foods are removed and then later reintroduced when symptoms have subsided. Foods that are to be avoided on FODMAP include dairy products, stone fruits (cherries, peaches, papayas, mangoes), cruciferous vegetables (broccoli, cabbage), legumes (beans, lentils), coffee and tea, onions, garlic, and wheat based products (bread, pastas, grains, cereals, crackers). FODMAP is a very restrictive diet that should only be done temporarily. Foods allowed on the FODMAP diet are meats, poultry, fish, seeds, fruits (bananas, berries, oranges, melon), specific vegetables (kale and cucumbers), and lactose free dairy products.

Specific Carbohydrates Diet

Specific carbohydrates diet is most similar to the gluten free diet, as it restricts a majority of carbs, especially added sugars and wheat products. Also excluded are potatoes, rice, and oats to limit the consumption of lactose and sucrose. Foods allowed on this regimen are lean meats, fish, aged cheese, dried or fresh fruit, nuts, natural dairy, honey or monosaccharides (glucose, fructose).

Low Oxalate Diet

Oxalates are substances found in plants and animals that form crystals from iron and calcium. Once formed in the body they're excreted through the urine, which involves the painful passing of kidney stones. To prevent this, the low oxalate diet is a regimen that eliminates foods high in oxalates. There are over 177 foods that contain oxalates, but there are levels graded from low to high that estimate the amount of oxalate in each food.

GAPS Diet

The GAPS (Gut and Psychology Syndrome) diet involves healing of the gut lining, especially with patients with digestive issues. This regimen involves two phases which are set up into six stages first followed by a full protocol for a longer period of time.

RESTRICTING foods from your kid's diet is one of the most effective ways to remedy issues that affect their gut and their mental well being. An elimination diet could be the solution that's necessary if your child is suffering from any issues within their digestive tract. Elimination diets separate problematic food groups from your diet in order to see how you react to them.

The main benefit is that by turning your reaction to certain foods you can pinpoint sensitivities and intolerances you may not have otherwise known about. Elimination diets are often more reliable and save considerable amounts of money when trying to evaluate food intolerances within a diet. Keep in mind that you may not figure out everything that you're sensitive to that causes your symptoms. Your plan should be strategically created to ensure the most common food allergens are eliminated. The commitment for a majority of these diets are 4 to 6 weeks if not longer, so keep that in mind. With allergies and tolerance out the way, we still focus on diets that could be of great importance for behavioral problems starting with GAPS in Chapter 5.

CHAPTER SUMMARY

The basic purpose of the elimination diet is to have foods that cause a food intolerance removed and later reintroduced to observe any possible symptoms. Implementing an elimination diet has been shown to provide benefits that could improve overall health when done correctly. Elimination diets have to be structured differently because each person has a genetic sequence that is distinct to one another. Although elimination diets are the best way to isolate food intolerance symptoms, there's a likelihood for becoming nutrient deficient.

The first part of the elimination diet is the removal phase, where the suspected foods are restricted from the diet for no longer than 3 weeks. Following this removal phase is the reintroduction, where the foods you eliminated are brought back into the diet gradually. Symptoms are observed for the next 3 days and recorded when possible. Some symptoms to look out for are joint pain, rashes on the skin, bloating, changes in breathing, headaches, trouble sleeping, fatigue, and changes in bowel habits. The basic elimination diet also removes milk, eggs, nuts, added sugars, citrus fruits, wheat, alcohol, shellfish, processed meats, soy, beef, and gluten.

In the next chapter you will learn about the GAPS diet and how it can be used to treat common behavior disorders such as ADHD and depression...

FIVE

GAPS Diet

In a 2011 study conducted by Dr Lidy M Pessler, it was shown that 64% of kids with ADHD symptoms saw improvements after being placed on a strict elimination diet. GAPS is one of the best-known diets to improve ASD, ADHD, and other conditions.

For kids' that are experiencing health problems, the GAP diet benefits these conditions by removing sources that cause the development of leaky gut. The culprit behind leaky gut is often foods with added sugars and gluten products, which are on the list to be avoided. These foods are replaced with fermented and whole foods rich in fiber that help repopulate the microbiome with healthy bacteria. For this reason, the GAP dieting emphasizes preparing homemade meals, as processed and junk foods from restaurants are also to be avoided with this regimen.

This diet has been linked with the treatment of other behavior related conditions such as tourettes, depression, and eating disorders. Because gut inflammation is associated with the diversity of the microbiota, use of the GAP diet is proactive with the formation of psychobiotics in the gut that can improve mental health and behavior patterns. Although research regarding elimination dieting protocols for behavior disorder treatment has been shown as effective for a large portion of studied children, further research is needed for conclusive evidence.

The true benefit of the diet has been the ability to steer children away from the bad habits of consuming excess sugar, bad fats, and artificial ingredients. Home cooked meals allow the opportunity for children to get involved with preparation of the food they'll be consuming. Kids will have a deeper understanding that toxins are unnecessary additives in foods when they experience cooking healthy, delicious meals with their family. The earlier kids are exposed to healthier eating lifestyles, the easier it is for them to form good habits for later on.

While there are good outcomes and results from the GAP diet, it comes with a few downsides as well. The foods allowed in the introductory phase of the diet are restricted to broths, soups, and probiotic foods. This phase of the diet lasts for a minimum of 1 year with small amounts of food being increased gradually, which may cause pangs of hunger or stomach discomfort as the diet continues. It is also possible that children in the midst of a growth spurt may experience nutritional deficiencies, as vitamins and minerals from a wide variety of foods are needed. With this protocol it's always to consult a doctor or nutritionist before proceeding with the diet.

The foods to be avoided in GAPS are grains, refined carbohydrates, pasteurized dairy, and starchy vegetables. Familiarization with the type of foods in each category will make eating on this regimen a lot easier.

Grains

This includes all conventional baked goods as well as pasta, cereal, biscuits, and crackers. These foods are restricted as they're likely to cause an inflammatory response in the gut lining.

Dairy

Only fermented dairy products are allowed to be consumed. Pasteurized milk and milk products contain antibiotics and hormones that can also affect the gut lining similarly to grains. The exception to dairy products allowed is butter.

Starchy Vegetables

The banned foods in this category are potatoes, sweet potatoes, yams, parsnips, as well as beans and legumes.

Refined Carbohydrates

These carbohydrates are specific to processed foods found in packaging. These include canned goods, ready made meals, processed meats, and candy.

Getting the body accustomed to the selection of foods takes a certain amount of time, depending on each individual. Toddlers and older children will have a challenging time adjusting to a diet that eliminates all processed sugary, starchy foods. If your kids are picky eaters, you'll want to skip the introductory phase and move straight to the Full GAP diet for a month or two. This phase is a little easier and will have them only consuming meat, fish, eggs, fermented vegetables, and cold pressed fruit juices. After the two month period they can transition to the introductory phase.

As the diet is very low in carbohydrates, it's normal to experience hunger pains for 1-2 weeks as the body transitions to becoming more fat adapted. Fat adaptation involves the breakdown of lipids instead of glucose for energy. Less sugar is being consumed as well, which will result in a large amount of bad bacteria dying off in the microbiota. This is a good outcome, but it can result in stomach upset, diarrhea, and cramping as the stomach adjusts.

GAPS Diet Phases

First Stage

Plenty of liquids are consumed at the beginning of the diet, with homemade meat stocks prepared between meals and at each meal. Using the stock that has been prepared, soups with meat and/or vegetables are served as well. Gradually small amounts of fermented vegetable juice can be added to meals, starting with 1 tablespoon and increasing up to 4-5 tablespoons per day. Homemade fermented dairy (sour cream, yogurt, whey) can be substituted if possible.

Second Stage

Continue with liquid meals of broth and soup. Add egg yolks to meals, starting with one soft boiled or raw/organic yolk per day to a bowl of soup. Increase this amount to 1 yolk per bowl of soup. Progress to a whole egg if no symptoms are presented. Meat stews or casseroles can be added as well. Increasing amounts of ghee butter should be implemented starting at 1 teaspoon a day.

Third Stage

Continue with hot liquids in the diet as in the second stage. Add avocado, cooked eggs, fermented vegetables, and seed/nut butters and flours. Seed and nuts should be soaked/sprouted, then dehydrated and ground for easier digestion. Use GAP approved, homemade nut/seed flour cooked with ghee or butter to make pancakes/waffles.

Fourth Stage

Hot liquids and probiotic foods are still consumed. Add roasted or grilled meats, cold pressed oils (olive and coconut), and fresh squeezed juices. Start with 2-3 tablespoons per day then progress to 1 cup. Start with an easier digestible juice like carrot, then progress to celery, cabbage, mint, parsley, and then beet. If no symptoms are present, a combination of the vegetable juices can be used. Baked goods from sprouted nuts/seeds can be added to the meals.

Fifth Stage

Staple foods are stocks, soups, probiotic foods, juices. Gradually add pureed cooked apples with honey. Start to introduce raw vegetables like lettuce or cucumbers. If no symptoms are noticed add carrots, onions, cabbage, bell peppers, and tomatoes. Vegetables must be chewed well to ease digestion.

Sixth Stage

Continue with staple food items (stocks, soups, probiotic foods, juices). Fresh stone fruits are added (peeled apples, peaches, apricots, cherries, mango, papaya) berries, tropical, and lastly citrus fruits. GAP approved baked goods can be added with honey or dried fruit as a sweetener.

Full GAPS Diet

The final sixth stage is a continuous phase that lasts anywhere from 1.5 to 2 years depending on the condition of the child. The day should start with a room temperature glass of water or fermented/regular vegetable juice. A majority of the foods should consist of stocks/broths, soups, meat, fish, eggs, fermented dairy, cooked/raw/fermented vegetables, and cold pressed fruit juices. The full GAPS diet also allows seasonings and spices back into meals; Celtic sea salt, Himalayan pink salt, ground rosemary/thyme, oregano, parsley, dried basil, cinnamon, bay leaf, black pepper, and nutmeg are all approved. GAP diet fruits are recommended between meals and bakcd goods with approved ingredients can be incorporated.

Reaching the last stage of the GAP diet also allows you to be a little creative with your meals while adding some more variety. The seasonings and salts introduced back in have great flavor and take these items to another level. These recipes are also great ideas to add vitamins and minerals into foods that are familiar with your kids:

<u>Chicken Liver Muffins</u>

Ingredients:

1 lb. of chicken liver (organic raw whole livers)

1 medium carrot

1 medium celery root (.4 lbs)

½ medium onion

1 clove garlic

1 large egg

¼ tsp black pepper

⅓ tsp sea salt

1 tsp lemon juice

½ tsp baking soda

½ tsp mustard powder (or creamy mustard)

Instructions:

1. Rinse livers in cold water and trim connective tissues as necessary.
2. Soak livers in a vinegar & water solution for 20 minutes to remove harsh taste (use 1-2 tsp apple cider vinegar).
3. Once soaked, rinse gently in cold water. Pat dry with a towel.

Mixing ingredients:

1. Add all ingredients (except baking soda and lemon juice) in a food processor and pulse until mixture resembles a muffin batter.
2. Do not overmix. If the mixture is too thin, you can add bread into the processor for a bulkier texture.
3. Before baking, add the baking soda and lemon to the mixture and give it a final stir with a spoon.

Bake the muffins:

1. Preheat the oven to 350F.
2. Transfer to a mini-muffin pan and bake at 350F for 15 minutes.
3. Once cooked, allow them to cool before removing from the pan. Muffins should have a spongy texture.

Avocado Egg Boats
Ingredients:
2 ripe avocados, halved and pitted
4 large eggs
Kosher salt
Freshly ground black pepper
3 slices of turkey bacon
Chopped chives (for garnish)
Instructions:

1. Preheat the oven to 350F. Scoop out 1 tbsp of avocado from each half. Discard or reserve for later use.

2. Place hollowed avocado halves on a baking tray. Crack eggs into a separate bowl, one at a time. Transfer one yolk to each avocado half, then spoon in egg white without spilling over.
3. Season with salt and pepper, then bake until whites are set and yokes are no longer runny. Est. time 20-25 minutes. (Cover with foil if avocados are beginning to brown.)
4. In a large skillet, cook turkey bacon until crisp and then transfer to a towel lined plate. Chop into small pieces on a cutting board.
5. Top avocados with bacon and chives before serving.

Chicken Soup
Ingredients:
2 lbs chicken meat
10 cups filtered water
2 medium carrots (diced)
2 celery stalks (diced)
1 large bell pepper (red or yellow, diced)
10 cauliflower florets (chopped)
4 oz. crushed tomatoes
1 medium onion (diced)
4 garlic cloves (minced)
1.5 tsp of lemon juice (fresh squeezed or apple cider vinegar)
2 bay leaves
1 tsp dried thyme
$\frac{1}{2}$ tsp. Black pepper
2 tsp. Celtic sea salt (or to taste)
2-4 tbsp of fresh herbs (for garnish)

Instructions:
Prepare and Cook the Chicken Meat & Bones

1. Wash the chicken, place in a deep pot and add the filtered water. Bring to a boil.
2. Once boiling, bring the stove to medium-low and spoon off foam or scum at the top of the water.
3. To the pot add bay leaves, black pepper, and thyme. Reduce heat and simmer for 20-30 minutes while you prepare the vegetables.

Prepare and Add the Vegetables

1. Clean, peel, and dice the carrots, onion, celery root, and celery stalks. Chop cauliflower florets and then finely dice. Add vegetables to pot and simmer for 20 minutes until tender.
2. Add crushed tomatoes, bell pepper, lemon juice, minced garlic, and salt. Simmer for 10 minutes then turn off heat. Adjust seasonings to taste if needed.
3. Add fresh herbs (parsley, dill, etc.). Allow chicken soup to sit in the pot for 20 minutes to cool before serving.

Beef Meatballs
Ingredients:
1 lb. ground beef (or minced meat of your preference combined with beef)
½ onion (red or white)
3 cloves of garlic

1 medium carrot
1 celery root (grated)
⅓ ground rosemary
⅓ paprika
¼ tsp of sea salt or Himalayan pink salt
Instructions:
Chop & Combine the Ingredients

1. Place vegetables in the processor and chop.
   Then add ground meat and spices and pulse
   until combined.

Shape the Meatballs

1. Scoop the meat from the bowl and form into 1-
   1 ½" balls. Place meatballs on a baker's sheet.
   You can also use a mini muffin pan, which gives
   the meatballs a nice crust from baking them in
   their own juices.

Bake the Meatballs

1. Bake at 400F for 20 minutes until the meatballs
   are no longer pink inside. For a crustier surface,
   bake at 420F.
2. Meatballs can be served in a creamy sauce to
   make them juicier and softer, along with a
   serving of gluten-free pasta.

PUMPKIN & Beetroot Salad

Salad ingredients:
3 cups of beetroot

3 cups of pumpkin or squash
½ cup of pumpkin seeds
1 avocado
Salad dressing ingredients:
1.5 tsps Dijon mustard (or brown)
1.5 tsps lemon juice
1.5 tsps sweetener (honey or maple syrup)
¼ tsp sea salt
1 tbsp chia seeds
Oil (optional)
Roast The Beets And Pumpkin:

1. Peel, cube, oil, salt & pepper the beetroots and pumpkin. Place on a baking sheet and bake for 25-35 minutes on 425F. They should turn out sweet and caramelized around the edges.

Prepare the Salad Dressing

1. While cooking the veggies, whisk all the salad dressing ingredients in a bowl and set aside.

Assemble the Salad

1. You can either mix the salad dressing with greens or drizzle the dressing on top when serving, depending on your preference.

Coming Off GAPS Diet

After evaluating digestion for at least 6 months, you can progress into the reintroduction phase. Over the next few months restricted foods are gradually added in combination with the staple foods on the GAP diet. This process will continue with starchy vegetables, grain, and beans, while monitoring for any digestive issues.

Research surrounding this issue connecting gut inflammation to mental disorder has been controversial, but the intention of the GAP diet is shown to be effective. Foods that cause discomfort or digestive problems are identified and eliminated through self evaluation and observation. Many of the foods that are restricted from the diet have been conclusive for causing imbalanced gut flora through an analysis of a multitude of studies. Inflammatory foods can become problematic for developing children and establish poor dieting habits that can persist well into adulthood.

Even though it's an adjustment to not eat certain foods for a while, the key is to focus on the foods that you can eat. The benefits of the diet is phenomenal as it gives you the ability to heal your kids from autism, learning disabilities, and other physical symptoms such as eczema, allergies, and other issues. GAPS is still very restrictive and you still could want to consider some less aggressive starters. We cover it in LOD in the following chapter...

CHAPTER SUMMARY

The GAP diet aids behavior conditions of ASD, ADHD by isolating and removing the culprits for leaky gut, sugar and gluten. These foods are replaced with fermented and whole foods rich in fiber that can repopulate the gut microbiome. The GAP diet steers kids away from the bad habits of consuming excess sugar, toxic fats, and artificial ingredients. Getting the body accustomed to the selection of foods takes a certain amount of time, depending on each individual. Toddlers and older children will have a challenging time adjusting to a diet that eliminates all processed sugary, starchy foods. The foods in the introductory phase of the diet are restricted to broths, soups, and probiotic foods. This phase lasts for 1 year and small amounts of food are gradually increased.

Because less sugar is being consumed, this will result in a large amount of bad bacteria dying in the gut. This could be a good outcome, as it's a sign that conditions are getting better and the gut biome is becoming more balanced. The final sixth stage is a continuous phase that lasts anywhere from 1.5 to 2 years depending on the condition of the child. Reaching the last stage of the GAP diet also allows you to be a little creative with your meals while adding some more variety with new recipe ideas. After evaluating digestion for at least 6 months, you can progress into the reintroduction phase. Restricted foods are then added slowly back into the diet.

In the next chapter you will learn about the impact of oxalates in the body and how a low oxalate diet can help resolve behavioral problems...

SIX

Low Oxalate Diet

While mainly focused on kidney stones, LOD could prove beneficial with behavioral problems if we make the assumption they could be arising or have symptoms increased for gut inflammation. Understanding that the gut/brain connection can be impacted by foreign substances that irritate the digestive tract, isolating oxalates may help alleviate this issue. It's not easy to remove oxalates from the diet, because oxalates are mostly molecules bound within healthy, nutrient dense plants.

Oxalates can be a problem with some people that develop symptoms including headaches, dizziness, urinary issues, brain fog, migraines, fibromyalgia, joint pain or stiffness, IBS and gut problems, or kidney stones. If there is a high concentration of oxalates in the body along with low levels of fluids in the urine, these oxalates bind with calcium deposits to form calcium oxalate stones. As the amount of crystals grows larger in number, they form larger stones known as kidney stones that are excreted from the kidneys. Low oxalate diets help prevent the formation of these stones by lowering this concentration to moderate levels.

Excess amounts of oxalates in the body are often common also with patients suffering from cystic fibrosis. Humans lack genes that can break down oxalates in our body, which makes us reliant on our gut biome to degrade oxalate. Certain species of bacteria prevent stone formation by producing specific enzymes that alter chemical pathways to degrade oxalate salts.

Cystic fibrosis patients suffer from excess mucus in the respiratory pathways that builds up and becomes sticky, caused by an inherited genetic defect. These patients usually receive large amounts of antibiotics, which can destroy the population of bacteria responsible for degrading oxalates from their system. A low oxalate diet could restore some of these healthy bacteria and ease cystic fibrosis symptoms.

Over time oxalate crystals are accumulated and dispersed throughout the body, especially in the thyroid gland. Oxalates are naturally *oxidants*, which create damage to cell membranes due to their composition of oxygen molecules. The body recognizes these oxalates as a potential threat and sends an autoimmune response to destroy these crystals, which in turn destroys the surrounding thyroid tissue. As the thyroid gland is highly permeable and has a constant supply of blood through the capillaries, oxalates collected there slowly destroy thyroid function.

For individuals that have symptoms of an underactive thyroid, also known as hypothyroidism, the higher concentration of oxalates in circulating blood could damage cells that produce crucial hormones. When not treated, hypothyroidism can cause obesity, joint pains, infertility, and heart disease. Infants with this condition can experience difficulty breathing, hoarse crying, a large protruding tongue, jaundice of the eyes and skin, and an umbilical hernia. Teenagers and young adults have signs of delayed puberty and teeth development, and poor mental advancement. Low oxalate diets can gradually lower oxalate concentration and allow the thyroid to properly heal. Consuming foods that are lower in oxalates will give the body time to remove oxalate buildup that has occurred over a period of time.

Oxalates also have a correlation to those diagnosed with autism. When researchers examined the oxalate levels of diagnosed children, oxalate concentration was 2.5 times greater within the urine samples and plasma concentration was three times greater. Autism has also been connected to seizure episodes, which is a known symptom of high oxalate concentration. Studies have shown that having high levels of oxalates, known as hyperoxaluria, could be involved in the direct pathology of ASD.

Compromised gut issues that are prevalent with autism could impair the ability to metabolize oxalates, as this affects how much oxalates from the diet is absorbed. Deficiency in a bacteria species oxalobacter formigenes have been shown to cause oxalate sensitivity, which disrupts the breakdown of oxalates in the gut. Conditions of ADHD have evaluated similar pathology with these individuals as well.

Adjusting to the low oxalate diet could be a lot easier than more restrictive diets because many of the foods can be moderated. High oxalate foods can be paired with foods containing significant amounts of calcium, such as dairy products. Contrarily, you can enjoy low oxalate foods that are present in a wide variety of food groups, from an assortment of meat to fruits.

To fall under the guidelines of a low oxalate diet, daily intake should be under 100mg, but suitably under 50mg.

It's possible to stay within this amount efficiently by sticking to low oxalate foods for most days of the week and rotating in high oxalate/calcium rich meals on occasion. Higher oxalate foods can also be rotated back into the diet when symptoms are alleviated and removed when sensitivities begin to reoccur.

These oxalates are present in numerous foods, so some may find it challenging to stay within the recommendation limits. Being a source of nutrients, limiting most plants from a diet can put you at risk for a deficiency that may require additional supplementation. Vegans and vegetarians that rely on particular plants for getting daily amounts of protein or fiber will face obstacles staying within 50mg without consuming meat products.

Healthy foods such as beets, carrots, kale, spinach, and eggplant are high oxalate sources that have to be substituted with cruciferous vegetables (cabbage and cauliflower) or tropical fruit (bananas, mangoes, or avocados). These foods are moderate in oxalates and can be consumed on occasion within 2-3 servings per day: grape juice, cranberry juice, orange juice, strawberries, liver, sardines, brown rice, onions, buttermilk, and ginger.

Besides dairy products, some other low oxalate foods include herbal teas, raisins, melons, lean meats, wild rice, pasta, white rice, cucumbers, and peas.

As mentioned earlier with vegans, LOD has deficiencies with limited available protein sources that are on the approved list. Not getting adequate amounts of protein can affect the body negatively and have symptoms such as getting sick often, delayed healing, lack of muscle growth, poor recovery, weak connective tissue, bone loss, low neurotransmitters, low hormones, low enzymes, inability to detox, and poor sleep. In extreme cases this can affect the skin, hair, and nails, altering the composition to a very hard or brittle texture.

The purpose of consuming protein is to get the building blocks of protein, which is amino acids. When you eat protein, the bonds between the amino acids are broken down at the stomach level, in the intestine, and then it's absorbed into the body. The purpose of amino acids is for muscle repair, neurotransmitter precursors, and biological proteins. Biological proteins are the enzymes that make energy, help you detoxify, and make body tissue. Poor protein intake on the low oxalate diet could affect kids that are currently growing, as low amino acids in the bloodstream is correlated with impaired bone length growth.

Obtaining the appropriate amount of fluids on the LOD is vital in preventing the formation of stones inside the kidneys. Recommended amounts of water intake have always been arbitrary, as there are inconsistencies for the amounts to consume. Urine output should be around 2-2.5 liters per day and some individuals may live in warmer climates where this output could be compromised. For these reasons, it's recommended that water is kept at 8-10 cups per day. Certain fluids should be avoided while on the diet, including water with added calcium supplements or cranberry juice. These beverages have extra amounts of calcium that will bind with the oxalates in the body to form crystals.

Diets that are low in calcium have a higher likelihood for the development of these crystals, which is why it's recommended to have several servings of calcium. 2-3 servings daily are good amounts to add if oxalates in your diet are in the range of 200-300mg. Yogurt, milk, and even ice cream are good sources for calcium intake to bind circulating oxalates in the body. Cheese can supplement calcium as well, although the sodium content should be considered when consuming it in large quantities.

Vitamin C has also been found to affect the levels of oxalates in the gut. A double-blind study was conducted with adults that formed calcium oxalate stones and non-stone forming adults, both of whom received 1 gram of vitamin C for 2 6-day phases. At the end of the phases urine samples detected increased levels of oxalates, indicating a strong association with the supplement and oxalate concentration. From this study it was concluded that vitamin C can be easily converted to oxalates in the gut, so it's wise to avoid supplementation if on a LOD.

Following this is as a guideline, in addition to drinking adequate amounts of water and boosting your intake of daily calcium should be enough to prevent calcium stones from forming in the kidneys. Avoid consuming high oxalate foods often and pair those foods with daily products when possible. There's also less risk for gut inflammation when this protocol is followed.

You can have success sticking to a low oxalate diet when you have an understanding of which foods have higher concentration than others. The key to the diet is to stay under the moderate amount of oxalate limit for the day, which would be 40-50mg. Food that's allowed and to be avoided on a LOD are grouped into four different categories based on their oxalate content: very high: more than 100mg per serving, high: 50-100mg per serving, *moderate:* 10-25mg per serving, low: 5-9 mg per serving.

Consuming foods that are in the low to moderate category are the best options for staying within the maximum limit for daily oxalate intake. These foods are still very satisfying and are great ingredients for recipes to make for your meal plan. Here are some of the foods you enjoy that are the lowest in oxalate concentration:

Fruits: bananas, blackberries, blueberries, cherries, strawberries, apples, apricots, lemons, peaches, watermelon

Vegetables: Mustard greens, broccoli, cabbage, cauliflower, mushrooms, onions, peas, squash, zucchini, artichokes, garlic, brussel sprouts, bell peppers, lettuce, chives, corn, chili peppers, cabbage, asparagus

Grains: white rice, corn flour, oat bran, wild rice

Protein: eggs, fish, poultry, meat

Dairy: yogurt, milk, cheese, butter

Beverages: coffee, water, fruit juice

Herbs & Spices: basil, chili powder, marjoram, nutmeg, onion powder, oregano, white pepper, sage, thyme, garlic powder, coriander, cinnamon, dill weed, horseradish, parsley

These are some of the foods that have moderate levels of oxalates that should be limited in daily servings:

Fruits: avocados, dates, kiwis, oranges, dried prunes, dried figs, grapefruit

Vegetables: carrots, kidney beans, olives, parsnips, boiled potatoes, sweet potatoes, fava beans

Grains: brown rice, quinoa, granola, Cream of Wheat, egg noodles, pasta

Protein: Tofu

Beverages: Black tea, carrot juice, lemonade, rice milk, soy milk, tomato juice

Herbs & Spices: black pepper, caraway seed, cloves, cumin seed, curry powder

Nuts: macadamia nuts, pistachios, walnuts

These items have the highest amount of oxalates of all the food groups and should be avoided when possible on the LOD:

Fruits: raspberries, canned pineapple, dried pineapple

Grains: whole wheat flour, cornmeal, wheat bran, grits

Vegetables: beets, navy beans, okra, baked potatoes, fried potatoes, collard greens, rhubarb, rutabaga, spinach, turnips, yams, soybeans

Beverages: hot chocolate

Herbs & Spices: poppy seed, turmeric

Nuts: cashews, hazelnuts, peanuts, almonds, and pecans

With an overview of the foods to consume and the ones to avoid, you can now start trying mixing up some ingredients to make some delicious recipes. These are a few of my favorites:

RED ONION & Mushroom Omelet

Ingredients:

4 eggs

2 cloves of garlic

½ green bell pepper

½ red onion (finely chopped)

8 button mushrooms (sliced)

Salt & pepper to taste

Instructions:

1. Add 1-2 tbsp of cooking oil to a pan to medium heat on the stove. Add red onion, green pepper, and garlic. Saute until soft and fragrant. Add sliced mushrooms and cook for 3-5 minutes until they soften and shrink. Remove from heat and set aside.
2. Whisk eggs with salt and pepper, then add to the heated pan. Add sauteed mushrooms and vegetables on top of the egg mixture. Make sure to add sautee right after eggs so they stick to the omelet.
3. Flip omelet and finish on pan for 30 seconds before serving.

EGG ROLL in a Bowl

Ingredients:

2 tsp sesame oil
1 lb of ground chicken
14oz coleslaw mix
8 oz white mushrooms (sliced)
4 cloves of garlic (chopped & divided)
4 green onion stalks (whites & greens separated)
2 tbsp white vinegar
2 tbsp Braggs Amino Acid (soy sauce alternative)
1 tbsp fresh ginger grated
1 lime
1 tbsp Sriracha (or another hot sauce)
1 tbsp cornstarch
¾ cup fried wonton strips

Instructions:

1. In a large sized skillet, heat 1 tsp of sesame oil over medium high heat. Add chicken and cook until browned.
2. Add coleslaw mix, mushrooms, garlic, and white parts of green onion. Cook until cabbage is tender, about 10 minutes.
3. Meanwhile, prepare sauce. Whisk vinegar, soy sauce, ginger, and juice from ½ of the lime, sriracha, and cornstarch together.
4. Add sauce to chicken and cabbage mixture. Cook 1-2 minutes until well combined.
5. Serve garnished with green parts of green onion, lime wedges, and 2 tbsp of fried wonton strips per serving. Serve over rice if desired.

PANZANELLA TOSCANA
Ingredients:

3 tbsp olive oil

4 cups sourdough bread (1" cubes)

2 large tomatoes

1 cucumber (1" chunks)

1 yellow bell pepper (1" chunks)

1 red bell pepper (1" chunks)

½ red onion (1" chunks)

20 fresh basil leaves (roughly chopped)

3 tbsps white or red vinegar

2 cloves of garlic

3 tbsps of capers

½ tsp black pepper

½ cup of olive oil

1 tsp of dijon mustard

Instructions:

1. Preheat the oven to 375F. Drizzle 3 tablespoons of olive oil over bread cubes and place on a baking sheet. Bake about 10 minutes until the bread is toasted and slightly browned. Set bread cubes aside.
2. Place cucumbers, tomatoes, cucumber, bell pepper, red onion, basil, and capers in a large salad bowl.
3. Whisk garlic, mustard, vinegar, olive oil, and black pepper together.
4. Add bread and dressing to the salad bowl. Toss to combine. Let it sit at least 10 minutes to soak up some of the dressing.

BLT WRAPS

Ingredients:

10 cherry tomatoes

1 cup shredded cheddar cheese

1 lb. turkey or beef bacon (1" pieces, chopped)

½ head of butter lettuce

Instructions:

1. Cook chopped turkey or beef bacon in a skillet and brown on both sides. Drain and set aside.
2. Halve the cherry tomatoes. Add ¼ cup cheddar cheese to each lettuce leaf, then add ¼ cooked bacon and cherry tomatoes on top.
3. Roll the wraps up before cutting them in half.

BANANA MUFFINS

Ingredients:

4 lightly beaten eggs

4 mashed ripe bananas

2 tbsp vanilla extract

3 tbsp maple syrup

½ tsp salt

1 tsp baking powder

½ cup of coconut flour

½ tsp baking soda

Instructions:

1. Preheat the oven to 325F and proceed to grease the muffin pan.

2. Next, mix eggs, vanilla extract, maple syrup, and banana in a bowl until evenly combined.
3. In a separate bowl, add coconut flour, baking soda, baking powder, and salt. Mix until combined. Pour dry components into wet ingredients and mix until they combine evenly.
4. Let the dough sit outside for 5 minutes before dividing it into the muffin tin. Place into the oven for 20 minutes, checking periodically when finished with a clean toothpick.

WHEN A HIGH CONCENTRATION of oxalates are present in the body, this can cause a host of problems for those with existing physical and mental conditions. Finding what can help to manage this problem is half the battle, as there's a wide variety of foods that contain oxalates and preparing a proper meal is crucial to remove them from the body.

Furthermore, gut dysbiosis or low calcium supplementation can increase the buildup of oxalates, which can create a host of symptoms until further addressed. By evaluating any signs of these symptoms, you can reverse these effects by implementing a low oxalate diet to correct the build up and find the root cause of any issues that you may be experiencing. Transitioning from a moderate level of oxalates to lower levels is the best method to adjust to a diet that is this restrictive of healthy food options. While there are irrefutable reports of LOD being used successfully to reduce behavioral problems in kids, we move to elimination diets designed for kids with ADHD in the next chapter.

. . .

CHAPTER SUMMARY

High concentrations of oxalates in the body with low fluid levels in the urine can lead to calcium binding with the oxalates to form kidney stones. Humans lack genes that can break down oxalates in the body, which makes us reliant on our gut biome to degrade oxalate. Following the protocol of a low oxalate diet can help minimize oxalates in our diet and eventually remove buildup from the body. To fall under the guidelines of a low oxalate diet, daily intake should be under 100mg, preferably under 50mg. Diets that are lower in calcium have a higher likelihood of the development of these crystals; it's recommended to get 2-3 servings of calcium daily. There's a wide variety of foods that contain oxalates and preparing the correct meals are crucial to removing them from the body.

Obtaining the correct amounts of fluids on the low oxalate diet is also vital in preventing the forming of stones within the kidneys. Consuming foods that are the low to moderate category are the best options for staying within the maximum limit for daily oxalate intake. You can have success sticking to a low oxalate diet when you have an understanding of which foods are high in oxalate concentration compared to other foods

In the next chapter you will learn about a diet modification strategy to deal with food intolerances and behavior disorders with kids...

SEVEN

Feingold and FAILSAFE

L ow salicylate diets are designed to treat **ADHD** symptoms, but have shown results for other conditions too. These elimination diets can be used as diagnostics in food intolerance and treatment when successfully introduced. Diet modification has been shown to be an essential strategy for resolving behavior problems in children with numerous clinical studies. The association between diet and behavior has been established with trials of various elimination diets. Many of these diets also counterbalance problems of gut inflammation, which is why a further look into the Feingold or FAILSAFE regimen may prove beneficial for parents looking for alternative solutions for their kids.

By now you may be familiar with some of the leading causes of food intolerance and behavior affliction that plague many of our children, however the few mentioned are related to natural chemicals known as salicylates. The FAILSAFE protocol (Free of Additives, Low in Salicylates, Amines and Flavor Enhancers) and Feingold diet focuses on removing these compounds from the diet to reduce the adverse reactions from susceptible individuals. In the 1950s, scientists discovered that over-the-counter aspirins that contained salicylates worsened skin irritations and allergies in those that had food intolerance. With research conducted over the next couple of decades, it was discovered that these compounds were also present in natural foods that were assumed to be otherwise healthy.

Eliminating salicylates from the diets of those suffering from food intolerance also alleviated other symptoms that were observed. One clinical trial followed diagnosed children with hyperactivity on the FAILSAFE diet to monitor improvements in behavior. Kids that improved behavior were given challenges to reintroduce foods that were eliminated at the start of the diet and were observed again by their parents. With the exception of four children, the parents all reported that their kids showed signs of ADHD. From this study it could now be concluded that removing foods with natural or chemical additives is beneficial.

Eating salicylates in moderation can help, especially if you're not processing them properly.

Additive chemicals can also have a negative impact on the moods of those that are food intolerant. Similarly to the kids in the study diagnosed with ADHD, children that participated in an elimination diet recorded adverse feelings after consuming particular foods that were reintroduced. Symptoms ranged from suicidal thoughts, depression, inability to focus, melancholy, lethargy, shakes, inability to sleep, and becoming argumentative. Even after the administration of psychotropic drugs to relieve mood disorders, removing additives have proven to be more effective with patients once culprit foods were identified.

Low salicylate diets can also improve physical conditions that affect the skin. Individuals that suffer from eczema usually deal with this condition for a prolonged amount of time, with very little success from prescribed treatment. In fact, some of these products contain a solution known as salicylic acid, which can make problems even worse for those that are sensitive. When these products are used symptoms of hives, rashes, and skin swelling can occur. Avoiding salicylates that are ingested or used topically is the best way to prevent these conditions.

Removing salicylates from the diet can also have positive changes on sleep patterns. Side effects of these compounds include insomnia, difficulty falling asleep, frequent waking up, waking up too early, sleep walking, vivid dreams or nightmares, and restless legs. When initiating an elimination diet for children experiencing one of these symptoms, it's common to receive feedback from parents that sleep patterns have returned to normal. Getting infants and toddlers to fall asleep can involve lots of trial and error after many tiresome nights before recognizing that the problems are originating from the diet.

This elimination regimen seems like the perfect solution for identifying a sensitivity that afflicts children and adults alike with numerous symptoms, but this diet has some consequences. Both Feingold and FAILSAFE diets have been controversial since their origin because of their restriction of nutrient dense foods. These diets involve very lengthy time periods for evaluation and the risk of developing a deficiency is possible the longer they're continued. Children may become frustrated with the limited options and share food with friends or eat restricted foods unconsciously. It can become difficult for parents to force their kids to eat specific foods against their will, particularly if they have symptoms of ADHD.

For parents that find making lifestyle changes a bit uncomfortable, these diets will be a challenge to get used to. It may take you up to six months to implement these diets because many times spouses aren't supportive of any diet change, but it does get easier once you get used to it. You have to substitute large portions of food in the pantry and the refrigerator to provide what's needed for your child's nutrition. Doing so will require some financial obligations and a few weeks to adjust to the food bill costs for finding alternatives to foods you're accustomed to purchasing. As you further commit to these diets, this bill should decrease as there will be more banned foods that are unnecessary or will become undesirable to you or your child. You will also need more time to prepare meals to avoid most of the banned ingredients that would be found in restaurants or processed foods at the grocery.

Feingold

The introduction to this diet starts with the removal of all artificial additives that could lead to behavioral issues: artificial colorings and flavorings, preservatives, sweeteners, and foods containing salicylates. Reactions from salicylates can be very similar to that of dyes, so often the kids that have strong reactions to dyes are the same kids that have a reaction to salicylates because they're a form of salicylates. Eliminating fruits and vegetables is a big hurdle for many to overcome when considering the Feingold diet because a majority of people grew up believing and being told that fruits and vegetables are good for us. They are needed in our diet, so you'll learn how to remove these foods from your diet and eliminate those food sensitivities. Next, after removing foods with salicylates, reintroduce them to the diet and monitor for any physical symptoms. If symptoms occur then the salicylates are removed permanently and kept on the banned foods list.

If there is a sensitivity to salicylates, you're likely to

encounter a food or a prepared meal outside of your home that will cause you to express symptoms if not precautious. On this list are the foods/substances that should be avoided when possible:

Aspirin, preservatives (BHT, BHA, TBHQ), artificial colors (blue 1 &2, green 3, orange B, red 2, 3, & 40, yellow 5 & 6), artificial flavorings (vanilla, peppermint, strawberry, raspberry), artificial sweeteners (aspartame, acesulfame-K, saccharin, sucralose), synthetic pesticides, and perfumes/fragrances

Aspirin

Aspirin is known for its pain relief properties and can alleviate fevers. It's salicylic acid causes health problems for people with sensitivities, which include skin irritation, rashes, hives, nasal congestion, headaches, nausea, stomach pain, and swelling of the hands and feet

Preservatives

BHT, BHA, TBHQ are preservatives that are frequently found in pastries and pantry shelf items that extend their freshness much longer than normal. BHA is banned in certain countries because research shows that it reacts with other ingested substances to cause the formation of carcinogens.

Both BHA and BHT are toxic to the liver and kidneys. BHA and BHT were originally developed as preservatives for petroleum. In the 1950s they were approved for the use in food products, which are now used to preserve fats and oils commonly used in crackers and pastry items. TBHQ is another chemical derived from petroleum and is a form of butane. TBHQ is being used more often since jurisdictions have placed more bans on trans fats. In order to preserve the foods and extend their shelf life, food manufacturers are using TBHQ instead. Consumptions of these additives, especially in higher doses, can result in allergic reactions, asthma symptoms, or anaphylaxis.

Artificial Colorings

These are coloring agents that are present in many sports drinks, confectionary accessories, condiments, seasonings, and processed foods/meals. Intake of these additives can heighten symptoms of children with hyperactivity and create carcinogenic compounds when digested in the body. Some of the potential effects of these coloring dyes are organ damage, asthma, headaches, cancer, birth defects, allergic reactions, hyperactivity, and behavioral problems. In kids the prominent effects seen are hyperactivity and behavioral issues, such as inability to concentrate, constant motion, disruptive behaviors, excessive talking, aggression, excessive touching, irritability, and meltdowns. These chemicals can also cause physical issues such as difficulty sleeping, nightmares, headaches, stomachaches, hives, asthma, daytime and nighttime wetting, motor and vocal tics, and more.

The use of food dyes has increased 500% since the 1950s. The FDA has a limit on the amount of carcinogens that's allowed to be used in one individual dye, but there are no guidelines on the total amount of these products to consume each day. There are no studies that have been done on the long term effects of ingesting dyes.

Many medications used to treat ADHD contain dyes, which can cause the very same symptoms you're trying to eradicate. You can ask your doctor to write a prescription for medicine without dyes. You can also transfer the contents of a dyed capsule into a clear veggie cap which can be found at your local health food store.

Artificial Sweeteners

Artificial sweeteners are substitutes for sugars that originate from the byproduct of various chemical compounds.

These sweeteners can alter gut microbial metabolic pathways, which can create inflammation and immune problems at some point. They are also linked with Alzheimer's disease, multiple sclerosis, autism, Parkinson's, chronic fatigue syndrome, and certain cancers. They can be found in most 'sugar-free' labeled products.

Perfumes/Fragrances

A 'fragrance' can be classified as hundreds of different chemicals for one particular ingredient, many which are not labeled on the product packaging. One of these chemicals could be phthalates, which are solvents used to make the fragrances last longer and reach deeper into the skin. Unfortunately, phthalates have been linked to autism and ADHD due to exposure in the womb. *Benzyl salicylates* that are found in most fragrances function similarly to phthalates and can cause allergic reactions to people with skin sensitivity.

AFTER REMOVING these substances for a period of time, it's possible for some people to reintroduce them to their diet slowly. The Feingold diet is shown to be effective after 4-6 weeks, which may be enough time to clear symptoms that we noticed before starting. However, some people will have to stay in the first phase of the diet for the rest of their lives because they're body has shown sensitivity to these foods.

The Feingold diet is helpful for this because they will research all the ingredients and find out if salicylates are used within the ingredients, such as with natural flavors listed in various products. If you have a child that is struggling with ADHD, Feingold should be your first step. So many kids with ADHD react to dyes and salicylates. Before moving on to bigger, more expensive protocols, Feingold should be tried first. Feingold is ideal for those that have made no dietary changes or are just eating the standard American diet because Feingold will provide which foods are without the additives, which makes your life a little easier. The substances that are removed temporarily are foods with salicylate and medicines that contain salicylates as well.

FAILSAFE

The elimination diet is set up in two parts; stage 1, where the body is cleansed completely from food chemicals and stage 2, the challenge phase. Stage 2 lasts much longer than the first because food additives are tested one by one to monitor for symptoms. If you consume a banned food during the elimination phase of the diet, you must wait and watch for symptoms for 3 days before starting over.

Elimination Phase

Start off by finding out what foods you can and cannot have before you go shopping for groceries. Check all the labels in the pantry for the substances mentioned on the list that are to be avoided. Next, choose a start date, keeping in mind the engagements that will be coming up over the following several weeks. To plan ahead further, create a meal plan of the foods that you'll be consuming including snacks that will keep you satisfied. When you're shopping for your new groceries, plan extra time for this shopping trip as you'll be reading labels more thoroughly this time.

Keep 2 diaries for recording your experiences; one for daily experiences and another for recording symptoms that you're experiencing. As you get closer to days 4 or 5 of the diet you'll mostly experience some symptoms of withdrawal from the familiar foods. You should start to see improvements after 2 weeks, which at that point you can proceed onto the next phase. If symptoms persist in 3 weeks, you may need to make an adjustment or extend the elimination phase for another week. Being symptom-free is important in order to move onto the next phase.

Challenge Phase

This is where you slowly challenge your system by slowly reintroducing certain foods back into the diet. To do it you need to consume the food for 7 days and then monitor symptoms carefully for the next 3 days. It would be wise to choose from a big food group like salicylates so that you add a wider variety of foods back to your diet earlier. The challenge food should be at a minimum of 6 servings unless otherwise indicated. For example, a cup for a serving of food should be consumed six times that day for 3 consecutive days to complete the challenge.

Mini challenges do not work as the chemicals may take time and repeated ingestion to see a significant response. Stick to the recommended serving amounts. It takes 3 days to see a reaction from food additives, 7 for salicylates and amines, and up to 10 days for milk. Next, wait until you've been completely symptom free for 3 days before starting the next challenge. This is important so that the recorded results are most accurate.

What to Avoid

Foods that are particularly strong smelling or tasting and environmentally unsafe substances are those that should be avoided on the failsafe diet. Some of these are listed here:

Artificial Food Additives: These include artificial colors, flavors, preservatives and antioxidants

Salicylates: Including polyphenols that are contained in natural whole foods (natural flavors, colors, and preservatives)

Neurotransmitters: all glutamates (especially MSG) and

amines (dopamine, serotonin, phenylethylamine, tyramine) which are found in aged meats and fermented cheeses

Aromatic Chemicals: fragrances and salicylates found in perfumes, air fresheners, cleaning products, cosmetics, menthol oral care products, and scented toiletries

Pharmaceutical Drugs: aspirin, ibuprofen, decongestant drugs, and anti-inflammatory creams all contain additives

IT'S evident that Feingold and FAILSAFE are two elimination diets that isolated the issues of behavioral health years before the epidemic seen in kids today. Both of these protocols are methods that can be used if using a full elimination diet is not an option for your child. Because salicylates are present in a wide variety of foods and consumer products, if you don't exclude all the chemicals the diet won't work. If you exclude everything from the start, the diet will be too difficult.

Following the guidelines listed is the key to getting good results while executing either one of these diets. Practicing patience will help you and your kids make the adjustments necessary to see positive changes. Expect shopping to become a more diligent process and your child to get accustomed to not eating some of the foods they enjoy. Reassure them that they'll have these restricted foods after a short period of time. Journaling also makes the process much easier because you can notice the change in effects while looking back. If you keep the food log long enough, you'll start to notice obvious patterns, so keep track of symptoms, behaviors, and illnesses in the order that you're seeing them throughout the day next to the foods that have been eaten.

While studies have been conducted that shows these protocols can work with a large portion of children, conclusive evidence that matches against pharmaceutical intervention has yet to tackle this issue once and for all. Eliminating 80% or more of the standard diet will bring its share of controversy with nutritionists but the results speak for themselves. With two prominent ADD and ADHD diets behind us, we switch focus to candida and its impact on kid's behavior in Chapter 8.

CHAPTER SUMMARY

One of the leading causes of food intolerance and behavior affliction is related to the presence of salicylates. Low salicylate diets can improve the physical conditions that affect the skin. The FAILSAFE and Feingold diets are controversial because they restrict nutrient dense foods and very lengthy periods of time for the evaluation of symptoms. Be prepared for the dietary lifestyle changes and financial obligations needed to adjust towards these diets beforehand. You will also need to dedicate more time to preparing food at home to avoid the list of banned foods and additives on these diets. The Feingold diet is shown to be effective at 4-6 weeks to clear any symptoms.

The first stage of the FAILSAFE diet starts with the elimination of all the foods that are on the restricted list. To successfully execute this, you need to follow a weekly meal plan for your approved foods and give yourself extra time to shop for the groceries that you need. Keep two journals to keep track of the symptoms that you're experiencing while on the diet. If symptoms do not persist after 2 weeks, you can move onto the next phase.

During the second phase of the FAILSAFE, slowly reintroduce foods back into your diet by consuming a minimum of 6 servings of the item for 7 consecutive days. Following the 7 days, carefully monitor for any symptoms for 3 days before moving on to the next food group. Artificial food additives, salicylates, neurotransmitters, aromatic chemicals, pharmaceutical chemicals are the substances that should be avoided while on the FAILSAFE diet.

In the next chapter you will learn about one of the leading causes for infection and mental health disturbances that originates in the lining of the gut...

EIGHT

Candida For Kids

W hile easier to track down and detect, candida has been discovered to cause similar behavioral conditions in kids. A small yet significant percentage of kids are even misdiagnosed as autistic while having severe candida yeast infections. Without understanding some of the true causes of existing behavior symptoms, a lot of time can pass as the condition continues to get worse.

Candida can be tricky to isolate because symptoms of this infection are similar to other illnesses that can occur in the body. It's been established that the gut/brain connection is essential and our microbiome is what provides our overall health. To maintain that health, it's important to learn about why these imbalances may occur inside of you, the impact of this infection on the brain, and what could be done to prevent it from happening to your kids.

Recognizing the signs and symptoms of an overgrowth is one of the most proactive ways to guage an infection. This overgrowth can create many problems which are noticeable and specific to the candida fungus that resides in the digestive tract:

Skin/Nail Fungal Infection:

Your skin and nails are good markers for what's happening inside your body. When nails are infected, noticeable traits are increased thickness, dry or cracked nails, ragged appearance or fungal infection in skin around the nail, cracked appearance, toenail discoloration (yellow, white, or black), and pain sensitivity.

Chronic Fatigue Syndrome:

CFS is a condition that is identified with extreme fatigue and paired with other symptoms of aches, pains, memory loss, and cognitive dysfunction. Chronic fatigue may be an occurrence from brain inflammation from the administration of antibiotics. Fatigue is frequently misdiagnosed as a psychological or a complex problem, for which other prescriptions are used to treat it.

Digestive Issues:

Candida overgrowth causes a significant amount of damage in the digestive tract and can worsen if not intervened expeditiously. As yeast growth proliferates it creates noticeable discomfort that will greatly affect daily living experiences. Some symptoms are GERD (acid reflux), bloating, craving sweets, itching, flatulence, diarrhea, beer belly, constipation, and higher triglyceride levels.

Skin Issues:

This type of skin infection often occurs in moist, warm areas of the body where fungi are likely to repopulate. Infections are seen in the groin and armpits, with candida being the most common cause of infant diaper rash. Other areas that infection can be noticed are at the corners of the mouth. Skin rashes can also present red, itchy patches known as psoriasis. When the immune system overreacts to an infection, this can result in a breakout of hives, indicating that the fungi is out of balance with good gut flora. Toxins released from candida yeast can also cause red, flaky *eczema* rashes to appear on the skin.

Depression and anxiety:

A majority of the neurotransmitters that affect our moods are produced in the gut by good bacteria. When candida yeast overgrowth occurs, this offsets our balance of good to bad bacteria and causes less serotonin to be secreted. Low serotonin levels place individuals at risk for developing anxiety and depression. Candida also releases toxic byproducts that negatively affect mental health. These toxins from the candida cells can be released into our circulatory system and trigger immune responses that cause irritability and mood swings.

ONCE THE SYMPTOMS for candida have been identified in a patient, a sample is collected for evaluation from the labs for results. Stool is inspected for discolored components of mucus, froth or foam, a white or yellow string like substance, or loose stool indicative of diarrhea. Oral testing for candida can vary from either a throat swab or the use of saliva, a concentrated oral rinse, or a mucosal biopsy.

HOW CANDIDA AFFECTS KIDS' **Behavior**

Many of the markers for mental disorders in children have been a misdiagnosis of candida overgrowth infection. Mental health has a strong link to the function of the gut biome, however medical professionals often remedy symptoms with interventions that create more problems. If testimonials are received from patients complaining of painful bloating, upset stomach, or an acid reflux, they're promptly given antibiotics that kill the bacteria in the gut. When the friendly bacteria population is lowered, yeast overgrowth becomes worse and the original symptoms for candida worsen.

Behavioral problems are a symptom of the antibiotics because friendly bacteria are responsible for the digestion of specific foods into compounds. Without the assistance of the bacteria these foods can create issues in the body. Candida yeast proliferation in the gut can lead to the production of toxic amounts of sugar, which blocks centers in the brain responsible for attention and speech. The infection also causes cravings for sugar, which feeds the fungi population and perpetuates a negative feedback loop that can only be resolved through dietary intervention.

CANDIDA DIET

The candida diet is a treatment option for individuals suffering from an overgrowth of the fungi in their digestive tract. The diet eliminates foods that encourage fungi population growth which include sugar, gluten, alcohol, certain dairy products and encourages low-sugar fruits, non-starchy vegetables, healthy fats, lean protein, and gluten-free foods Administering probiotics and some antifungals help repopulate the gut with friendly bacteria. Avoiding inflammation is one of the key protocols of the Candida diet, which prohibits the consumption of processed foods and caffeinated drinks are kept to a minimum.

Candida Cleanse

A candida cleanse is a precursor before the start of the diet that removes toxins from the body and clears out the digestive tract. The cleanse prepares yourself mentally for the discipline needed to restrict to a specific set of foods that you'll be consuming. Some side effects could occur like fatigue, headaches, mood swings, or changes in sleeping patterns. To start the cleanse you have two options: liquids only or cooked/raw vegetables. If you opt for liquids you can use either lemon water or bone broth. Cooked vegetables can be steamed or salads can be consumed with a small amount of protein at each meal.

The cleanse generally only takes a few days to complete, afterwards you can slowly start the candida diet by following the guidelines. Instead of removing sugar, caffeine, and gluten from the diet all at once, remove one at a time to avoid any symptoms of withdrawal or adverse reactions. These changes should be done over a time period of 2 to 3 weeks, if symptoms are mild then you can remove them sooner from your diet. If your kids are switching from caffeinated soda to fresh drinking water, gradually increase the glasses per day one at a time until they're getting the recommended amounts of water daily.

FOODS TO AVOID

The candida diet recommends avoiding foods with natural and added sugars, processed foods, some dairy products, refined grains, and many oils:

Grains: wheat, rye, spelt, barley.

Sweets and Sweeteners: sugar, honey, maple syrup, chocolate, molasses, corn syrup, agave, and artificial sweeteners.

Fruits: bananas, dates, figs, grapes, mango, and raisins.

Processed Meats & Fish: processed meat, swordfish, shellfish, tuna.

Dairy: cheese, milk, cream.

Condiments: ketchup, mayonnaise, barbeque sauce, soy sauce, vinegar.

Processed Oils: canola, soybean, fake 'butter' spreads, margarine, sunflower.

FOODS TO EAT

Low-Sugar Fruits: avocado, lemon, lime, olives.

Non Starchy Vegetables: artichokes, broccoli, asparagus, cabbage, cauliflower, celery, cucumber, eggplant, rutabaga, spinach, garlic (raw), kale, tomatoes, zucchini, and onions.

Non-Glutenous Grains: buckwheat, millet, oat bran, quinoa, teff.

Healthy Proteins: anchovies, chicken, herring, salmon (wild caught), sardines, turkey, eggs.

Dairy: ghee, yogurt, kefir, butter, yogurt (probiotic).

Low-Mold Nuts & Seeds: almonds, coconut, flaxseeds, hazelnuts, sunflower seeds.

Herbs, Spices & Condiments: apple cider vinegar, basil, black pepper, cinnamon, cloves, coconut aminos, paprika, rosemary, dill, garlic, ginger, oregano, paprika, rosemary, salt, thyme, turmeric.

Drinks: chicory root, tea, filtered water.

Non-Sugar Sweeteners: xylitol, erythritol, stevia.

Healthy Fats & Oil: extra virgin olive oil, coconut oil, sesame seed oil, flaxseed oil.

Fermented Foods: kefir, sauerkraut, olives, yogurt.

CANDIDA YEAST INFECTION has been identified as the one the main causes behind various physical symptoms and mental disorders in adults and children . This fungal dysbiosis of the gut needs proper dietary intervention to resolve the issue, otherwise health conditions can worsen. Inflammation and toxins produced by candida yeast eventually alter hormone levels in the body, which can have a major influence on modifying mood and behavior in children.

Avoiding foods that cause pathogens to become problematic in the digestive tract is sensible, since it conserves friendly bacteria of the gut flora while destroying the more unfavorable microbes. You have to make drastic dietary lifestyle changes in the body in order to fix an issue like this where there would be toxins present that can worsen the situation. Candida cleansing diet is a short-term diet solution and should be treated as such. Still, its restrictive nature emphasizes the need for supplements just as much as the previously mentioned diets.

CHAPTER SUMMARY

Candida can be tricky to isolate because symptoms of this infection can be similar to other illnesses in the body. Recognizing the signs and symptoms of an overgrowth is one of the most proactive ways to guage an infection. Many of the markers for mental disorders have been misdiagnosis of candida overgrowth infection. The candida diet is a treatment option for individuals suffering from an overgrowth of fungi in the digestive tract. The foods that are avoided are sugar, gluten, alcohol, and certain dairy products.

When the friendly bacteria population is lowered, yeast overgrowth becomes worse and the original symptoms for candida worsen. The candida cleanse is a precursor that's done before the diet to remove toxins from the body and to get yourself mentally prepared for the restricted set of foods that you'll be consuming. Behavioral problems are a symptom of the antibiotics because friendly bacteria are responsible for the digestion of specific foods into compounds. Also keep in mind that if you remove all banned food items for the diet all at once, you may face withdrawal or adverse reaction symptoms. Remove food groups once at a time within a 2 week period.

In the next chapter you will learn about the food supplements that may be necessary to compliment the restrictive nature of elimination diets...

NINE

Food Supplementation

I n this chapter, we discuss food supplements and how they can ease the process with elimination diets. Many much needed ingredients for your kid's growth could be affected and this could be a way around it. Removing known toxins from a diet comes with the risks of experiencing deficiencies from the lack of consuming essential vitamins and minerals. When you account for the soil degradation that occurs from industry farming practices and the increased presence of GMO foods in supermarkets, eliminating nutritious foods from diets almost seems haphazard.

Food intolerance is a complicated issue that should require the intervention of nutrition counseling for a practical solution. Kids' food intolerance is complicated because they need an accurate diagnosis in order to treat them properly. A dietary intervention with the inclusion of supplements could be the one solution that resolves these ongoing issues for good. Supplements can be beneficial if they're convenient for the person taking them and can effectively fill the void within your nutrition plan.

. . .

GROWTH DANGERS **With Elimination Diets**

Elimination diets can help parents identify the allergens and intolerances that negatively affect their kid's health. This method is highly effective for diagnosing issues, however it can be difficult to differentiate the signs of a nutrient deficiency and the symptoms of a food intolerance before it's too late. A 2017 study of 284 on elimination diets indicated that the parents reported a lower quality of life in comparison to parents of children with sickle cell disease or intestinal failure. The study showed that parents were able to identify foods that lowered the quality of life for their children, but were unable to stop what was causing their children's health to worsen.

Challenging foods on an elimination diet can become risky because symptoms observed during this lengthy phase (much like with the GAPS protocol) could be the sign of a nutritional deficiency. If nothing is done to correct the deficiency, the symptoms will persist and the issue will never correct itself because the nutrient dense food is banned from the diet. This can be observed with prepubescent children and their rapid growth spurts in adolescent years. Prohibiting dairy on an elimination diet may create a calcium deficiency in the body, if other foods rich in calcium are also removed from the diet as well. Consulting a nutritionist may be the best measure to take, especially if a lot of time and effort has already been invested into this diet.

WHAT SUPPLEMENTATION CAN DO

It's important to consume the proper amount of essential nutrients each day by consuming a wide variety of foods, however supplements can take their place if some nutritious foods are not available. Vitamins D and K can aid building strong healthy bones by supplementing them into your diet. Omega-3s are also essential for the nervous system and protection of the neuron cells in the brain, which can be obtained from cod liver oil pills or concentrate available in a variety of stores.

Supplements can be effective and beneficial for getting what's missing back into our diet, but you should use these aids with precaution. Vitamins can have many complications with certain medications and should be disclosed beforehand if you or your child are administered by a medical professional. Some vitamins counteract with blood thinners, chemotherapy drugs, and can make other drugs less effective.

Manufacturers also fortify their foods with vitamins and minerals within the recommended daily allowance (RDA) guidelines. Supplementing may put you well over the RDA that's required and cause the occurrence of side effects if not monitored. Excess levels of vitamin A can cause headaches, liver damage, reduced bone strength, and birth defects. High levels of iron causes nausea, vomiting, and can put you at risk for liver damage. Caution is advised for pregnant women, nursing mothers, and young children using supplements because many products have not been tested for safety and efficacy.

PROBIOTIC SUPPLEMENTS

Probiotics are often used as an intervention to reintroduce good bacteria back into the gut after having a microbe imbalance. Probiotics can be found in fermented foods, but is often available over the counter as a pill supplement. Many people find these supplements are more convenient because they can pick specific strains or culture 'concentrations' that have differing amounts of microbe populations. Probiotics can provide huge benefits by helping to digest food, keeping bad bacteria from getting out of control, creating vitamins, preventing leaky gut from occurring, and breaking down and absorbing medications.

Supplementation of probiotics is not the only way to get access to them, many of these good bacteria live in foods that we can ferment for consumption later. Fermented foods such as yogurt, carrots, pickles, kimchi, and sauerkraut can be made and eaten with meals for a healthy probiotic supplement. Besides foods, probiotics can be found in beverages, pills, powder, and liquids. To boost their effectiveness, they can be taken with a prebiotic that will feed your good bacteria and balance the gut flora.

CALCIUM

With dairy crossed off the list of most elimination diets as a calcium source, it's important to find an alternative source. Most parents are not aware that their children have needs for minerals in their diet and that deficiencies can cause problems when they're older. Calcium is one of the minerals that's needed to build strong bones. Older children need higher amounts of calcium, with up to 4 servings per day and infants needing about 700mg or 2 servings per day. Non-dairy sources for calcium include calcium fortified liquids: rice milk, goat milk, and orange juice. Additional options are cooked dried white beans, dried figs, spinach, oranges, sweet potatoes, tofu, sardines, salmon, instant oatmeal, and broccoli.

Some individuals have difficulty accessing some other alternative calcium rich foods and may opt for calcium supplements as a replacement. While this can be an option for some, supplements are not recommended for everyone. People with conditions of hypercalcemia have high levels of calcium in the blood and are at risk of kidney stones, kidney failure, and bone loss. Hypercalcemia is diagnosed by a blood test and can evaluate whether a calcium supplement should be recommended for you or not.

There also has been a link between calcium and heart disease, specifically coronary artery calcification which leads to atherosclerosis. When calcium and vitamin D are consumed in the diet, vitamin D takes the calcium from the stomach and concentrates it into the blood. From the blood, vitamin F takes it into the soft tissues, joints, and bones. Without having this essential vitamin from your diet, excess calcium can start to accumulate in the artery walls as a form of plaquing known as calcification. A CT scan can be used to monitor your CAC (coronary artery calcium) score to gauge if you're at low or high risk for a cardiovascular event.

Calcium carbonate is the most common source for calcium supplements on the market and often recommended by doctors for patients. This chemical compound is a form of rock that's found in eggshells and limestone. These calcium supplements could be a risk for older individuals or individuals with alkaline pH levels in the stomach and blood, as this creates difficulties in absorbing this mineral. Calcium is an alkaline mineral and if the pH of the body's fluid is not acidic enough, the excess calcium starts to build up inside the body. Not absorbing calcium properly causes it to be stored on the bones, within the eyes (cataracts), on the nerves (twitching and cramps), joints (tendinitis, heel spurs), kidneys (kidney stones), gallbladder (bladder stones).

Taking calcium citrate is the best supplement for absorption of calcium in the body, especially for individuals that have low acidic pH or digestive issues. It's advised to take your calcium citrate on an empty stomach, consuming the RDA dose recommended for your appropriate age range. Healthy vitamin F intake can be sourced from unsaturated fats in fatty fish (sardines or cod) or flaxseed oil to help absorb excess calcium in the blood.

Protein

Elimination diets such as the low oxalate diet can be restrictive with sources of protein, which can cause deficiencies. This can be especially impactful for vegetarians and vegans that source many of their foods from plants, nuts, and seeds. Because their diets already have restrictions on animal products, they will have to supplement protein from sources that have the essential amino acids needed for exercising and maintaining muscle.

There are nine amino acids that the body cannot produce and that must come from the diet. A source of protein is said to be 'complete' when these amino acids are all available in equal amounts. Some of these diets are better suitable to proteins that are sourced from plants: rice, pea, soy, and hemp. As a good source of essential amino acid within its profile (especially hemp), these proteins can be substituted out for animal products if necessary:

Soy

Many other plants don't have the nutritional value that soy does. As an option for vegans and vegetarians, it provides one of the best sources of essential aminos and is very efficient due to cost. In addition to higher levels of protein amongst other plant based supplements, soy protein also has plenty of B vitamins, zinc, vitamin D, and antioxidants in them as well. For every 100g, there's 36g of protein, 20g of fat, and 30g of carbohydrates on average.

The highest quality of soy to purchase is soy isolate, because of its high bioavailability. This means that the body will use a majority of what is digested. The next best is soy concentrate that has all of the sugars removed and the fiber content left behind, which is good for your friendly bacteria. Soy concentrates can be found in baked goods, meat substitute products, beer, and certain cereals.

The other type of soy is textured based protein (TVP), that's made from soy concentrate and found in most meat-based foods, such as curries, soups, and good stews.

Hemp

In addition to being a complete protein, it also has plenty of omega-3s and fiber that can easily provide satiety after meals. One 3-tablespoon serving has 15g of protein and 8g of fiber. Hemp protein contains more amino acids than soy protein, but less lysine than other proteins. Compared to other proteins, hemp is easier to digest because the aminos are readily available for absorption, such as edistin and albumin.

Pea

This legume-based protein is made by isolating the protein in yellow peas. The starch and fiber is then removed from the protein. Two scoops of the powder supplement is about 27g of protein and very little carbs in ratio to the serving size. Peas do contain a substance called purines, which converts to uric acid in the body and could create an inflammatory response in some people.

Pea protein also may not be digestible for everyone, due to the high content of fiber within each serving. For these individuals, there's still the option to purchase a hydrolyzed pea protein, which breaks down amino acids into smaller amounts to make digestion much easier. Plant based sources for protein should still be used with caution as many brands have been tested for high rates of arsenic and lead contamination. This is mainly due to the soil quality that the crops were harvested in.

<u>Rice</u>

Protein from rice is made by grinding up the rice grains and treating them with an enzyme that separates the starch from the protein. The advantage with rice protein is that it's very slow digesting and no carbs are included. The vital amino acid leucine that's necessary for muscle building is actually absorbed faster in rice protein than animal based protein like whey. Whey protein in comparison has more leucine but extra carbohydrates included into their servings. Rice protein is similar to pea protein where it's almost completely balanced with the amino acids except for one: lysine. Pea proteins are missing one essential amino acid as well, which is why pea and rice proteins are usually combined together by plant based supplement companies.

If using rice protein, always check the ingredients label for arsenic compounds being used in the processing of the product. Most of the contamination comes from the irrigation water to the grains and rice absorbs more arsenic than other food crops.

VITAMINS AND MINERALS

Fruits and vegetables are usually the primary source for obtaining vitamins in a healthy diet, however for individuals dealing with food intolerance this is not always an option. For this reason, vitamins fulfill their purpose as a useful aid, however relying on vitamins routinely is not the best solution either. Nutrients are activated from different components within the food once they are digested within the body, unlike supplement vitamins that are consumed isolated from one another. Vitamins also do not have any phytochemicals, which prevents oxidation, inflammation, allergy aggregation, bone loss, the formation of cancerous cells, and many other benefits.

Taking vitamin and mineral supplements was designed as a short term measure to address the problems of an inadequate diet. For a permanent resolution to a vitamin deficiency issue, it's much healthier to adopt a healthy lifestyle with the counsel of a dietician or nutrition specialist. These advisors can help with a proper evaluation of your situation and prevent incorrect dosing or interaction with any supplements that's not necessary.

It's easy to become an advocate for vitamin supplements if you're bombarded with health information about the topic. Belief that vitamins are a miracle cure for ailments or that they can be taken to prevent disease is a myth that has been debunked. Many companies see studies in lab animals or cell cultures and claim that these results will translate to human beings. The only way that scientists can verify that something works is if it is a randomized controlled study where some of the subjects achieved these miraculous results.

Using vitamins in this matter will result in major disappointment and is even risky to be taken without evaluation. Since vitamins interact with other vitamins and coenzymes in the body, taking a vitamin for one ailment can push the body out of homeostasis or overall balance. For example, the form of the vitamins and minerals in multivitamins aren't bioavailable and they're likely not in the correct natural ratios. Bioavailability indicates if the nutrients are being properly absorbed. When too much of one vitamin is present, this can be toxic and cause several health problems such as weakening of the teeth, blood clotting, high blood pressure, abdominal pain, diarrhea, cramps, sensitivity to light, nausea, skin lesions, neurological issues, and even death. Fat soluble vitamins (A,D,E, and K) are liable to become more toxic as they accumulate in the body's tissues because of their composition.

Vitamin recommendations also tend to differ in different countries, which can cause problems for individuals who are prone to overexposure to numerous vitamins present in their diets. For example, the United States recommends 1200mg per day for calcium, the United Kingdom recommends 700mg, and the World Health Organization suggests 500mg. Most manufacturers across the world are trying to comply with the recommended daily amounts for their specific nation and the RDAs aren't necessarily correct. Without evaluating your own blood work for deficiencies, these suggestions can create a toxic buildup of different vitamins that may not have been necessary in the first place.

The testing of these drugs is also not regulated, so the results of these studies for hyped supplements are not based on solid evidence. These companies can use cheap ingredients, contaminate the product with toxins, or include the wrong dosages on the packaging. Essentially, 97% of the supplements in the health food market are toxic, ineffective or both according to the Journal of the American Nutraceutical Association. Regulatory bodies such as Organics Consumer Association ensure that higher quality, organic products are labeled with NOS (Naturally Occuring Standard).

Fillers and binding agents are included in non-organic vitamin supplements because it allows the tablets and pills to be produced on a large scale. Some of these additives are not listed on the label at all. The manufacturers of big name brands are owned by pharmaceutical companies that often repackage their products into store brand names for discounted prices. These cheap vitamins have fillers that add weight to the product, tricking consumers that assume the heavier bottles have better quality. Value shopping for vitamins comes with a risk when looking for supplements for your diet.

The largest source of toxins in vitamins are GMOs that save money and require lower certification standards for manufacturers. These include almost all sweeteners such as high fructose corn syrup, maltodextrin, sucrose, and products derived from GMO corn. Ascorbic acid in the form of vitamin C is also derived from corn that is highly processed and laden with the chemicals that are used to extract the product in the facilities. Other toxins that are commonly used are magnesium stearate, carrageenan, titanium dioxide, methylcellulose, natural flavors, sodium benzoate, starch, povidone, carnauba wax, propylene glycol, acrylamides, benzoic acid, crospovidone, shellac, natural flavors (hidden MSGs), sorbitol, silica, laureth sulfate, and potassium sorbate.

For children, administration of vitamins can also be even more problematic. Vitamins marketed to kids have the appeal to appear as candy, which can cause kids to overindulge in consuming them if they're taken without discretion. Many multivitamins such as these have imbalanced ratios of ingredients that are not specific for the needs of individuals supplementing with them. These pills also have additives that could be dangerous if taken at high levels, such as biotin, kava, artificial coloring, polyvinyl alcohol, BHT, and talc.

Along with the toxins that are included into these low-grade vitamins is the packaging that contains them. Tablets are assembled by pressing composites of the vitamin together using binding agents and glues with high levels of heat, all which are harmful to long term health.

Consuming tablets regularly bio-accumulates chemicals that cause absorption problems and other symptoms in the body. Gelatin capsules are also problematic, as these are made of animal products that were fed antibiotics, preservatives, hormones, and chemicals that coagulate when digested in the intestinal tract. Time release capsules are made with hydrogenated oils (trans fats) that delay the release of the vitamin or mineral according to the time period listed on the label. These are one of the many ways trans fats have been snuck back onto the shelves despite being banned for consumer use in recent years.

Ironically, supplementing with some of these vitamins will most likely reintroduce many of the substances that you were trying to restrict with the various elimination diets. Many of these vitamin manufacturers are not regulated and interests are favorable towards profits instead of health. There's a time and place to use vitamins and minerals supplements, but use some precaution. It's better to take supplementation when you have full disclosure of all the foods you're consuming and an evaluation of blood work to monitor deficiencies.

The reason why is because there's a big difference between synthetic and natural vitamins. Natural vitamins offer higher quality because there is a different orientation and come in a complex of other vitamins. Trace minerals, cofactors, and enzymes are all incorporated and can replicate the effects of vitamins from whole foods. One way to tell the difference between synthetic and natural food vitamin complexes is to read the ingredients on the back of the bottle. The label will indicate if the product is herb based or a concentrated food, rather than a RDA percentage number that's the same for all the items listed. Nature has varied concentration of molecules within a vitamin complex.

Vitamins and minerals are a lot more effective when they're interdependent of each other, isolating individual supplements to aid your health is not how nature works and neither does your body. The most important thing to understand is when you add something in your diet, there is almost always some form of negative. Even with healthy food, your body is using energy and enzymes to digest it. When you start adding dozens of synthetic molecules in the form of vitamins there should be justification for doing so. Obtaining appropriate levels of nutrients on an elimination diet is a challenge, but you have to do a thorough research for vitamin brands that offer true quality.

The best products to purchase for long term use are those that are all-natural, non-synthetic, whole food supplements enclosed in vegetable capsules. The manufacturer should have a thorough background in sourcing raw ingredients and preferably should have an ISO standard or certified by NSF, which is regularly approved by sports leagues, dietitians, and coaches across the world for safe use. If there are supplements that you want to try that's not certified, you can investigate the products online at www. consumerlab.com or www.toxinless.com. These sites allow you to look at customer reviews or ask reviewers preliminary questions that have a comprehensive outlook about products currently on the market.

Synthetic vitamins can be used for a detoxification protocol or for a short term basis, it should never be used for maintenance in a lifestyle diet. These vitamins can be beneficial to push toxins out the body, but when consumed for longer periods of time can become toxic themselves. Synthetic vitamins can cause deficiencies in other nutrients because cofactors that are active in the product may cause imbalances in the body. These vitamins are artificial fractions of parts of vitamins that are produced from petroleum oil, coal tar, sulfuric acid, and cornstarch. A 2015 review of twenty years of research from the American Association for Cancer Research found increased risk of cancer in vitamin users over those who did not take any supplements. Oftentimes, these studies were linked to subjects that consumed synthetic vitamins for long periods of time rather than from natural whole food concentrates.

CHAPTER SUMMARY

Food intolerance is a complicated issue that should require the intervention of nutrition counseling for a practical solution. The various elimination diets introduced by parents can identify the allergens and intolerances that negatively affect their kid's health. Challenging foods on an elimination diet can also become risky because symptoms observed during this lengthy phase could be the sign of a nutritional deficiency. Probiotics are often used as an intervention to reintroduce good bacteria back into the gut after having a microbe imbalance.

Most parents are not aware that their children have needs for minerals in their diet and that deficiencies can cause problems when they're older. Calcium is one of the minerals that's needed to build strong bones and promote growth for adolescents. While this can be an option for some, supplements are not recommended for everyone. Elimination diets such as the low oxalate diet can be restrictive with sources of protein, which can cause deficiencies. This can be especially impactful for vegetarians and vegans that source many of their foods from plants, nuts, and seeds.

These fruits and vegetables are usually the primary source for obtaining vitamins in a healthy diet; however, for individuals dealing with food intolerance this is not always an option. For this reason vitamins fulfill their purpose as a useful aid, but relying on vitamins routinely is not the best solution either. The testing of these drugs are not regulated, so quality is poor in a majority of supplements that are currently on the market. Consumers should be diligent and research products with higher standards of quality than what is conventional offered.

Final Words

The lasting impact that food has on the body is convoluted, yet critical to understand. A large portion of the population does not recognize that problems originating from the gut are affecting their overall health and will need to be addressed at some point. The processes of what occurs inside our bodies can be explained simply enough for you to become proactive, yet many institutions and experts have given generic advice that's proven to be ineffective to transforming the public's health. When the health of adults continues towards a steady decline, so will the health of the kids in your household.

Children are being diagnosed with mental and behavioral disorders more often today than in past decades without acknowledgement of practical solutions for this epidemic. Naturopathic methods of treatment are viewed as controversial and many large studies are not given the funding needed to weigh comparative studies against the studies of orthodox medicine. Until there is a shift to the modern approach of dietary intervention to prevent disorders in children, we will continue to see these issues ongoing in the future.

It's understandable to see why certain dietary interventions are still controversial with kids, as it's very possible to create nutritional deficiencies with children whose bodies are still growing and developing. Disregarding the proper vitamins and minerals that's necessary for a well rounded diet can create worse problems than the symptoms caused by various elimination diets.

If a variety of foods are restricted in your diet, inclusion of dietary supplements that provide essential nutrients is a helpful way to overcome this problem. Harmful side effects from these supplements is always another risk, but it can be avoided by sticking to the recommended doses for your age range and closely monitoring your diet. It's very easy to have an imbalance of supplemental vitamins and minerals from the fortified foods and beverages that we consume regularly.

With my experience in this profession, I'm well aware of this potential for risk, but I know that alternative treatments with antipsychotics and stimulant prescription medications are very hazardous for our kid's health. In the long term these drugs never resolve underlying causes of behavior abnormalities and have side effects that create additional problems.

The reasoning behind prescription treatment seems to be related to brain chemistry imbalance and genetic disorders, yet gut health is rarely discussed as a precursor for any of these conditions. Protocols such as elimination diets help us evaluate food intolerances, allergens, and dysbiosis problems that can be resolved by modifying the foods that an individual is consuming.

It's been shown that the gut's direct connection with

the brain influences mental health and friendly bacteria introduced in the digestive tract can make positive improvements to brain chemistry. Learning about 'good' and 'bad' bacteria in the gut, you now have a better understanding of what types of foods feed different microbes.

Foods rich in fiber content gives us satiety after consuming them within our meals and feeds the friendly gut bacteria, which in turn creates enzymes, vitamins, and proteins that benefit our health. Foods that are commonly found on the avoid list of elimination diets increases the population of unfriendly bacteria and creates dysfunction within the digestive tract and various organs throughout the body.

While you try to be careful of what foods you feed your kids in your household, the occasional decision to eat out at restaurants or other households could be a decision made in error. The preparation techniques, hygiene standards, and additives that are used in foods vary greatly from person to person and location to location. If you're trying to resolve symptoms or behavior disorders, this could be an area you might have overlooked. Cooking all of your meals is a requirement.

Preparing meals for your household will become a satisfying experience, as you know that you're doing what's best for your own well being and the health of your kids. The sheer amount of functions in the body that the gut controls are a blessing from God and should never be taken for granted with negligent eating. Disbelief in the aiding power that the gut provides is the precursor that leads to disease, ailments, and maladies that negatively affect your quality of life.

My mission with this book was to address the parents of kids that are dealing with these issues and to give reassurance with an alternative of solutions. No one knows what's better for your kids than yourself, and you can make the best decisions for them when you have true discernment regarding nutrition. Having a deeper understanding of nutrition improves the well being of your household and makes you a much better parent. When I got a grasp of this information for myself, I felt empowered to know that I could take action steps to change the health of my child for the long term. The test results that the doctors revealed to us didn't make a difference in the final outcome.

If you find that your child is not responding well psychologically or not interacting socially, there's relief knowing that you don't have to settle for a ADHD or autism diagnosis from a medical professional. Preparation with information from this book will help you to become a proactive and attuned parent that can evaluate your child's dietary needs as well as being a dietitian in the field.

I certainly hope the book helped you get a better understanding on how to overcome the initial challenges with elimination diets for behavioral problems. There is a great community for these online, but it's highly advisable that you consult a doctor/nutritionist before putting your kid on any diet. Feel free to take a minute and leave a review if this book has improved your comprehension of this great information!

Your Words Could Help Someone Else to Heal

You have everything you need to know to put yourself family on the path to a happier, healthier life… and you're in the perfect position to help someone else find theirs.

Simply by leaving your honest opinion of this book on Amazon, you'll help other people find the information they need to take control of their gut health and find their way to wellness again.

WANT TO HELP OTHERS?

Thank you so much for helping me spread the word. This knowledge is far too important to keep hidden away.